UCLEAR WEAPONS POSE A SERIOUS THREAT?

Helen Cothran, *Book Editor*

Bruce Glassman, *Vice President*
Bonnie Szumski, *Publisher*

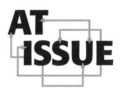

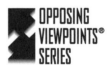

OPPOSING
VIEWPOINTS®
SERIES

GREENHAVEN PRESS
An imprint of Thomson Gale, a part of The Thomson Corporation

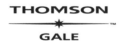

THOMSON
™
GALE

Detroit • New York • San Francisco • San Diego • New Haven, Conn.
Waterville, Maine • London • Munich

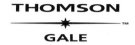

LIBRARY OF CONGRESS CATALOGING-IN-PUBLICATION DATA

Do nuclear weapons pose a serious threat? / Helen Cothran, book editor.
   p. cm. — (At issue)
Includes bibliographical references and index.
   ISBN 0-7377-2192-8 (lib. : alk. paper) — ISBN 0-7377-2193-6 (pbk. : alk. paper)
    1. Nuclear weapons. 2. World politics—Twenty-first century. 3. United States—Military policy. I. Cothran, Helen. II. At issue (San Diego, Calif.)
U264.D55 2005
355.8'25119—dc22   2004042533

Printed in the United States of America

Contents

Introduction

For over fifty years the "doomsday clock" has symbolized the threat that nuclear weapons pose to the world. The clock has appeared at various times on the cover of the *Bulletin of the Atomic Scientists*, a magazine about global security that was founded at the end of World War II by the scientists who developed the atomic bomb. Monitoring the clock is the responsibility of the *Bulletin*'s scientists and international affairs experts, who move its hands forward or backward depending on international events. When things go well, such as the signing of an arms control agreement, the hands move farther from midnight, which represents nuclear holocaust. When things go poorly, such as when a nation tests a nuclear weapon for the first time, the hands move closer to midnight.

On February 27, 2002, the clock's guardians moved the minute hand of the clock forward, from nine to seven minutes to midnight, only the third time in the history of the clock that the hand has moved forward. In explaining their decision, the *Bulletin*'s board of directors said that the September 11, 2001, terrorist attacks should have been a "global wake-up call" about serious threats to global security. Yet as *Bulletin* editor Linda Rothstein explains, "Even . . . after September 11, many of us—and much of the U.S. media—remain disturbingly disengaged from the rest of the world." The magazine's directors report that "moving the clock's hands at this time reflects our growing concern that the international community has hit the 'snooze' button rather than respond to the alarm." Moreover, although the September 11 attacks prompted the United States to wage a war against terrorism to reduce the chances that a terrorist group would attack America with weapons of mass destruction, many security experts argue that America is one of the main culprits making such an event likely to happen. Indeed, many analysts believe that America's actions—before and after September 11—have made the world less safe for all nations, including the United States.

Experts cite several key reasons why they have fingered America as a nuclear threat. To begin with, they point out, 95 percent of the world's thirty-one thousand nuclear weapons are located in the United States and Russia, with sixteen thousand of those operationally deployed. In addition, most of the U.S. weapons that have been removed from the active stockpile have not been dismantled but stored for possible future use. The United States will retain a stockpile of over ten thousand warheads well into the future.

Another fact that worries scientists and security experts is that U.S. weapons labs are now refining old weapons and designing new ones. For example, weapons scientists are designing "bunker busters," nuclear weapons designed to penetrate deeply buried targets in order to destroy weapons labs and storage facilities dug deep into the mountains of hostile nations. Many arms experts contend that building more nuclear

4

weapons—no matter what type—is simply fostering nuclear proliferation and further endangering global security.

The United States also continues to stockpile nearly 750 metric tons of weapon-grade uranium and 85 metric tons of weapon-grade plutonium. Since America has never satisfactorily kept track of these materials, many critics claim, it is impossible to verify if all of it is accounted for. Many commentators worry that some of this material may be migrating into the hands of terrorists, who could use it to build "dirty bombs," conventional explosives packed with nuclear materials that could be used against the United States.

Developments on the international front have experts worried as well. One of the most serious concerns is America's 2001 withdrawal from the 1972 Anti-Ballistic Missile (ABM) treaty, which prohibited the United States and Russia from developing space- and ground-based defensive nuclear weapons. The Bush administration believes that a missile defense system, capable of destroying enemy missiles in the air, is crucial to protect the U.S. homeland from nuclear attack; since the treaty did not allow America to develop such a system, the administration felt it necessary to quit the treaty. However, critics point out that the launching of a missile defense system will only encourage other nations to develop weapons to defeat it, leading to arms proliferation.

Another international diplomacy failure on the part of the United States, according to those concerned about global security, is President George W. Bush's provocative speech in which he named Iran, Iraq, and North Korea the "axis of evil" in part because of their attempts to develop nuclear weapons. Bush put these nations on notice that America would not sit idle while they pursued the development of weapons of mass destruction. Many commentators believe that this veiled threat will only force these nations and others to develop nuclear arms as protection against an aggressive America.

For these reasons the guardians of the doomsday clock insist that before they can move the hands of the clock farther from midnight, the United States must seriously reexamine its nuclear policies. The authors in *At Issue: Do Nuclear Weapons Pose a Serious Threat?* discuss the extent of the nuclear danger facing the world today and debate the best methods for enhancing nuclear security. The doomsday clock is a clear indicator that a reassessment of current nuclear dangers is vital. As *Bulletin* analysts put it, "The clock is ticking."

1

Nuclear Annihilation Is a Serious Threat

Robert S. McNamara and James G. Blight

Robert S. McNamara was secretary of defense to Presidents John F. Kennedy and Lyndon B. Johnson. James G. Blight is a professor of international relations at Brown University's Watson Institute for International Studies. They wrote Wilson's Ghost: Reducing the Risk of Conflict, Killing, and Catastrophe in the 21st Century.

During the Cold War the United States and the Soviet Union engaged in a nuclear arms race. More than ten years after the end of the Cold War, America and Russia still have enough nuclear warheads to virtually annihilate large sections of each other's populations. This policy of amassing nuclear missiles to deter attack is no longer morally justified. Today's nuclear weapons are so powerful that if used they could extinguish the entire human race.

For 40 years, we have lived with a situation so bizarre it is almost beyond belief.

Launch on warning

U.S. nuclear forces have been controlled by a "launch on warning" strategy. In order to reduce the number of our weapons that would be destroyed by a Russian first strike, our warheads stand ready to be launched while Russian warheads are in flight. No more than 15 minutes can elapse, under the policy, from the time of first warning of a Russian attack and the launching of our missiles, which means the president must evaluate the danger and decide whether or not to push the button with no time to study the situation.

To make that possible, the commander-in-chief of the U.S. Strategic Air Command carries with him a secure telephone, no matter where he goes, 24 hours a day, seven days a week, 365 days a year. This telephone is linked to the underground nuclear command post of the North American Aerospace Defense Command, deep inside Cheyenne Mountain in

Colorado, and to the president. The president, wherever he happens to be, always has at hand nuclear release codes in the "football," a briefcase carried for him by a U.S. military officer.

The standing orders of the commander of the strategic forces are that he must be able to answer the telephone by the end of the third ring. If it rings, and if he is informed that a nuclear attack of enemy ballistic missiles appears to be underway, he is allowed two to three minutes to decide whether the warning is valid (over the years, we have received many false warnings) and, if it is, to formulate his recommendation to the president. In the next 10 minutes, the president must be located and advised. He must discuss the situation with two or three of his closest advisors (presumably the secretary of defense and the chairman of the Joint Chiefs of Staff) and transmit his decision, along with the codes, to the launch sites.

The president's options would essentially be these: He could decide to ride out the attack and defer until later any decision to launch a retaliatory strike. Or he could order an immediate strike, thereby launching U.S. weapons that were targeted on military-industrial assets in Russia. The Russians presumably have analogous facilities and arrangements.

Nuclear extinction

The possibility of nuclear extinction is real. It exists today, this minute, despite the fact that the Cold War ended more than a decade ago. It is true that the U.S. and Russia have made substantial reductions in their arsenals since the late 1980s—between 1987 and 1998, the U.S. reduced its nuclear force from 13,600 strategic warheads to approximately 7,500, with the Soviet Union and Russia moving from 8,600 strategic warheads to about 6,450. Yet in terms of the security of the human race from nuclear holocaust, these reductions still leave the U.S. with the capacity to kill approximately 67 million Russians using only one-third of its forces, while the Russians can kill 75 million Americans, using 40% of their weapons. This assumes that each side's weapons are directed at military targets: Many more people could be killed, with far fewer weapons, if population centers were made the principal objective of an attack.

The possibility of nuclear extinction . . . exists today, this minute, despite the fact that the Cold War ended more than a decade ago.

Nuclear weapons blast, burn and irradiate with a speed and finality that is almost incomprehensible. This is exactly what the U.S. and Russia continue to threaten to do to one another with their nuclear weapons. It is useful to recall what happened when the U.S. dropped one atomic bomb each on Hiroshima and Nagasaki [Japan] in August 1945. These bombs had roughly one-twentieth of the destructive power of the average bomb in our arsenal today. In Hiroshima, approximately 200,000 died—men, women, and children. In Nagasaki, an estimated 100,000 died. On November 7, 1995, Itcho Ito, the mayor of Nagasaki, recalled in testimony to the International Court of Justice his memory of the attack:

"Nagasaki became a city of death where not even the sound of insects could be heard. After a while, countless men, women and children began to gather for a drink of water at the banks of the nearby Urakami River. Their hair and clothing scorched and their burnt skin hanging off in sheets like rags." Begging for help, they died one after another in the water or in heaps on the banks. The radiation began to take its toll, killing people like the scourge of death expanding in concentric circles from the hypocenter. Four months after the atomic bombing, 75,000 had suffered injuries, that is, two-thirds of the city's population had fallen victim to this calamity that came upon Nagasaki like a preview of the Apocalypse.

The threat to annihilate one another can no longer be morally justified.

Why did so many civilians have to die? The U.S. was seeking to end the war without having to fight its way to Tokyo, island by island, and the civilians, who made up nearly all of the victims in Hiroshima and Nagasaki, were unfortunately living and working near military targets. While their annihilation was not precisely the objective of those targeting the bombs, it was an inevitable result of the choice of those targets.

It is worth noting that at one point during the Cold War, the U.S. had more than 200 nuclear warheads targeted on Moscow, because it contained so many military targets and so much "industrial capacity." Presumably, the Russians similarly targeted many U.S. cities, because of the connection to its "military industrial capacity." The statement that our nuclear weapons do not target populations is totally misleading in the sense that the so-called "collateral damage" of our strikes would include tens of millions of Russians dead.

The U.S. and Russia no longer target specific missiles or other specific sites (although retargeting can be done in less than five minutes). But in other respects, very little has changed. Therein lies a great danger, one exacerbated by the lack of public awareness of it. Bruce G. Blair, a former U.S. Air Force nuclear-missile-launch officer who is now president of the Center for Defense Information in Washington, D.C., conducted in-depth interviews [in 2000] with officials at all levels of the U.S. nuclear command structure. From these interviews, Blair concluded that "The United States has about 2,200 strategic warheads on hair-trigger alert, according to Strategic Command officers. Virtually all missiles on land are ready for launch in two minutes, and those on four submarines—two in the Atlantic and two in the Pacific—are ready to launch on 15 minutes' notice, officers say."

Morally unjustified

Prior to the Soviet Union's dismantling, the threat to use nuclear weapons was conditionally justified, from a moral point of view, by the existence of a bitter Cold War between East and West. But that condition no longer exists. As Presidents George W. Bush and Vladimir V. Putin . . . proclaimed at their meeting in Slovenia [in 2001], the U.S. and Russia are no longer enemies. Yet we continue to threaten one another, and the entire human race, with nuclear extinction. Since the threat to annihilate one another can no longer be morally justified, it is time—past time—to move safely, steadily and verifiably to reduce the risk of nuclear catastrophe. Failure to do so is morally unacceptable, militarily unnecessary and extremely dangerous.

Will we continue to sleepwalk into a potential nuclear catastrophe? We hope not. Instead, it is our hope that nuclear catastrophe can be kept at bay until the work is accomplished—until nuclear weapons no longer exist. As a first step, but only a first step, we strongly endorse Bush's proposed unilateral reduction from the current level of 7,500 strategic nuclear warheads to approximately 1,500–2,500, and to remove the remaining weapons from hair-trigger alert.[1]

1. In 2002 the United States and Russia agreed to reduce the number of their warheads to the 1,700–2,200 range by 2012.

2

Nuclear Weapons Have Made the World Safer

C. Paul Robinson, interviewed by James Kitfield

C. Paul Robinson is director of Sandia National Laboratories; chairman of U.S. Strategic Command, which is in charge of U.S. nuclear weapons; and author of the white paper "Pursuing a New Nuclear Weapons Policy for the 21st Century." A physicist, Robinson headed the nuclear weapons program at Los Alamos National Laboratory for twenty years and was former president Ronald Reagan's chief negotiator and head of the U.S. delegation to the Nuclear Testing Talks in Geneva in the 1980s. James Kitfield is a correspondent with the National Journal.

Nuclear weapons have made the United States and its allies safer. America's enemies refuse to target the United States or its friends with biological or chemical weapons because they are afraid that American leaders will retaliate by dropping nuclear warheads on their countries. However, America should begin phasing out its most powerful nuclear weapons—which when dropped result in thousands of civilian casualties—and begin developing low-yield nuclear arms more suitable for targeting military bunkers, where leaders of rogue states make and store weapons.

National Journal: In a post–Cold War era when most policy makers are focusing on reducing nuclear arsenals, you argue in your paper ["Pursuing a New Nuclear Weapons Policy for the 21st Century"] that nuclear weapons not only "have an abiding place on the international scene," but also that new ones should be tailored for new kinds of deterrence.

C. Paul Robinson: As I wrote this paper, it felt like putting my head in a guillotine, because I knew that some people were going to try and chop it off for making these arguments. A lot has been done in recent years to delegitimize nuclear weapons to the point that I find people are lulled into a belief that nuclear weapons are going to go away soon, and thus we needn't worry about them anymore. But it's ridiculous to think that we can "uninvent" nuclear weapons.

I also happen to think that nuclear weapons have not only been vital to U.S. national security, but also that history has turned out better for our having nuclear weapons. U.S. nuclear weapons help maintain peace, and a lot of other nations depend on our nuclear umbrella. So, like it or not, for the foreseeable future we have no alternative but to continue to depend upon nuclear weapons and the deterrence they provide.

Nuclear weapons are legitimate

Are there no compelling strategic and moral arguments for, as you say, "delegitimizing" weapons of such horrific destructive potential? For instance, the United States signed the Nuclear Nonproliferation Treaty, which calls for non-nuclear states to forgo nuclear weapons, and for nuclear weapons states to work to reduce their arsenals eventually to zero.

The NPT Treaty, the arguments surrounding the Comprehensive Test Ban Treaty, and a lot of the rhetoric we heard from the Clinton White House all suggested that sooner or later nuclear weapons are going to go away. I simply don't believe that is true. I think it's important that people wake up and realize that nuclear weapons have meant a lot to our security, and we'd better make sure that our arsenal doesn't erode if our future depends on it.

And you've taken on the mission of sounding the alarm?

No one likes thinking the unthinkable, because it's a tough business. But someone's got to do it. I guess after spending my entire career in this field, I don't think anyone else knows more about the subject than me.

Nuclear weapons have not only been vital to U.S. national security, but also . . . history has turned out better for our having nuclear weapons.

Arms control advocates would argue that the NPT is largely responsible for many nuclear have-nots doing without nuclear weapons.

Yes and no. I believe the establishment of NATO [North Atlantic Treaty Organization] did more to prevent proliferation than the NPT, because it extended our nuclear umbrella over the nations of Western Europe that could relatively easily have developed their own nuclear weapons. I think there's a lesson in that example which applies today to South Asia.

The Bush Administration has proposed deep reductions in our offensive nuclear arsenal as a sweetener in selling its proposed national missile defense shield. At some point, might such reductions erode the United States' ability to extend its nuclear umbrella?

Different strategies

I support deep reductions, but at some point [those cuts] would call our umbrella into question. I worked on a report on that subject for the commander in chief of U.S. Strategic Command as a member of the Strategic Advisory Group. Essentially, our blueprint concluded that at some point between 2,000 and 1,000 nuclear weapons, we will run into speed bumps and probably a stop sign on reductions. It's not an exact science, and that level would still represent a dramatic reduction from today's massive U.S. and Russian nuclear arsenals.

At some point in reducing our arsenal, we also have to switch from bilateral to multilateral negotiations, because our nuclear arsenal has to deter a potential threat from unforeseen alliances that might develop in the future between other nuclear states. Stranger things have happened throughout history. Somewhat counterintuitively, a world in which there are just a few nuclear weapons would also be very dangerous, because the possibility that one side would "break out," and secretly construct a dominant nuclear force of a hundred or so weapons, would be quite high.

A world in which there are just a few nuclear weapons would . . . be very dangerous.

Do you think the Bush Administration's proposed missile defense system will lessen the need for some offensive nuclear weapons in the deterrence equation?

I believe both offensive and defensive systems can coexist as part of an overall national security policy, though I have yet to hear that policy articulated. You'll never have a defense, however, that is dominant against offensive nuclear weapons. When I speak publicly on the subject, I also ask audiences to consider that the United States or one of its allies were attacked with nuclear weapons one day, and our proposed missile defense system worked as advertised. Say only 5 or 10 percent, or whatever number you pick, of the attacking nuclear missiles got through. Do you really think the war is then over? . . .

Recently, Russia has threatened to rearm some of its ballistic missiles with multiple warheads if the United States unilaterally abrogates the Anti-Ballistic Missile Treaty in order to build a missile defense. Would that be a worrisome development?

When I heard [Russian president Vladimir] Putin talking about doing that, I knew we needed some new talking points with the Russians, because I can't think of anything more stupid. Presumably, we would be the target, since MIRVs [multiple independently targetable reentry vehicles] were built to attack missile fields. As the United States has gotten rid of most of our land-based missiles and decreased our reliance on that leg of the strategic triad, however, we no longer present those kinds of targets. Today we have roughly 800 ICBMs [intercontinental ballistic missiles], and we've telegraphed our intention of going down to below 500 land-based missiles, all with single warheads. So if MIRVs didn't make much sense in the first place, they make even less sense today.

The need for lower-yield nuclear weapons

In your paper, you argue that the United States needs to tailor its nuclear arsenal to deter new types of threats, especially chemical and biological weapons. Do we really need to find new uses for nuclear weapons?

Not necessarily new. We had a pretty good test case with Iraq during the [1991] Persian Gulf War. If you look at the volumes of chemical and biological weapons later reported by United Nations weapons inspectors, it was astounding what Iraq possessed. Why weren't those weapons of mass destruction used? Many military experts I've talked to are absolutely convinced it was because of a secret letter sent by President [George H.W.] Bush threatening the gravest consequences if such weapons were released. President [Bill] Clinton made a similar threat against North Korea during a crisis in 1994.

If our implicit threat of nuclear retaliation deterred rogue states such as Iraq and North Korea, why do we need new nuclear weapons?

The problem is, the strategic nuclear policy we developed during the Cold War has been stretched about as far as possible to fit a changing post–Cold War era. Today, we are threatened not only by nuclear weapons in the arsenal of peer nuclear competitors like Russia, but increasingly by biological, chemical, and radiological weapons that could kill huge numbers of people in a flash. Yet it's pretty incredible to think that the United States would respond to such an attack by vaporizing 11 million people in a rogue state just because they were poorly led. Where the hell are we going to use missiles with four to eight warheads, or half-megaton yields? Even the few "tactical" nuclear weapons that we have left have high yields of above 100 kilotons. I would hope a U.S. President would think it was crazy to use such weapons in response to a rogue-state attack.

After a decade of trying to sort out what we learned from the Cold War and how we might tailor our nuclear deterrence and deterrent message to fit the future, I now argue that we need lower-yield nuclear weapons that could hold at risk only a rogue state's leadership and tools of aggression with some level of confidence.

We need lower-yield nuclear weapons that could hold at risk only a rogue state's leadership and tools of aggression.

Isn't the United States' vaunted conventional military superiority—based in large part on our increasingly accurate precision-guided weapons—enough of a deterrent?

No. We've seen examples as recently as the [1999] air war with Serbia, when we attacked underground targets with conventional weapons with very little effect. It just takes far too many aircraft sorties and conventional weapons to give you any confidence that you can take out underground bunkers. By putting a nuclear warhead on one of those weapons instead of high explosives, you would multiply the explosive power by a factor of more than a million.

Wouldn't fielding new, low-yield nuclear weapons capable of penetrating underground bunkers require new designs and a return to nuclear testing?

In my paper, I conclude that we would neither have to conduct testing nor redesign for such a weapon, because we have them already. Right now, all of our weapons have primary and secondary stages. Through a process known as "boosting," you get a thermonuclear reaction. The primary alone, however, has a yield of 10 kilotons or less, or basically what you would want for a bunker-buster or a weapon that would cause relatively low collateral damage. All we have to do is send these weapons back to the factory and replace the secondary stage with a dummy. The beauty of that approach is that we are already very good at building dummy secondary stages. For safety and costs reasons, most of the weapons we have flown and tested in the past have had dummy secondary stages. So we could develop these lower-yield weapons without forcing the nuclear testing issue back onto the table, with a richer database of past tests, and at relatively low cost.

We need to carefully think through our posture of nuclear deterrence.

On the issue of nuclear weapons tests, the Bush Administration caused a furor when it was reported that they instructed the nuclear labs to develop a streamlined plan for a return to testing.

I read those stories that jumped to the conclusion that the Bush Administration was planning a return to nuclear testing, and that's wrong. There was a congressionally mandated commission, however, that recently looked at why it would take the nuclear labs roughly two years to return to testing. If we discovered a serious problem with the nuclear stockpile, the commission members suggested to me that a President would probably drop-kick me out of the Oval Office if I said it would take us two years to figure out what was wrong. You simply can't have people who stay up at night worrying about the security of the nation kept in doubt for that long. So, the Bush Administration has asked that we go back and study the issue to figure out why it would take so long and how we might streamline a resumption of testing. We haven't come up with the answers yet.

During the 1999 debate over the Comprehensive Test Ban Treaty, you expressed considerable skepticism over the ability of the Department of Energy's Stockpile Stewardship program to ensure the long-term reliability and safety of the nuclear stockpile without testing. Has anything happened in the interim to change your thinking?

You're the first person to ask me that. I would say that since 1999, the Stockpile Stewardship program has, if anything, surprised me by working a little bit better than I would have anticipated. I still have my reservations, however, about whether the program can substitute for testing over the long term. In my mind, the jury is still out on that question. As long as our reliance on a nuclear deterrent is crucial, we'll be taking a chance until we know for certain that Stockpile Stewardship is a reliable, long-term substitute for testing.

Are you seriously worried that aging will cause a catastrophic defect in our nuclear stockpile?

The toughest single thing I've had to do in my entire life was phone the commander in chief of Strategic Command and inform him that we had identified a problem with a particular warhead that affected a significant portion of the stockpile. We had to retarget many of our weapons and work like hell to figure out a fix. Our system of confidentiality proved itself in that instance, because we kept it all very, very secret. But that is one phone call I hope no one ever has to make again, because it was very, very tough.

How do you respond to critics who believe that by tailoring new nuclear weapons for new types of deterrence, you would make their eventual use in a crisis more likely?

My response is that for God's sake, then, let's think this through in advance rather than doing it on the fly. Say Iraq had instigated the first use of biological or chemical weapons during the Persian Gulf War, causing huge numbers of casualties. How would we have retaliated to make good on President Bush's threat? By vaporizing 11 million people? Because I can tell you, we haven't given a lot of thought to this issue. We need to carefully think through our posture of nuclear deterrence, because whatever decision is made during the next crisis will leave a message to all of history.

Why not send a message that the United States will not be the first to use nuclear weapons?

The burden is on those who believe it is immoral to threaten nuclear retaliation for the use of chemical or biological weapons to propose an alternative. I subscribe to the advice of [former British prime minister] Winston Churchill: "Be careful above all things not to let go of the atomic weapon until you are sure, and more sure than sure, that other means of preserving the peace are in your hands." Those words reflect my thinking on the subject very well.

3

Nuclear Weapons in the Hands of Terrorists Pose a Serious Threat

Jeffrey Kluger

Jeffrey Kluger is a senior writer for Time *magazine.*

The proliferation of nuclear materials, especially from the former Soviet states, has enabled terrorists to obtain uranium and other bomb-making materials with disturbing ease. While weapons-grade uranium is difficult to obtain, lower-grade radioactive rubbish, which can be used to make conventional weapons that spew radiation when exploded, is plentiful. Smugglers are transporting nuclear materials along well-established drug routes in Europe and successfully evading border authorities.

The six men who gathered at the roadside cafe southeast of Moscow [in December 2001] did not go there for the food. They went there for the uranium. Some of the men, members of the Balashikha criminal gang, claimed to be in possession of 2 lbs. of uranium 235, the kind of top-shelf radioactive material that can be used to build weapons. They were asking $30,000 for the deadly merchandise. The others—the buyers—seemed prepared to pay it. The deal may actually have gone off had Russian security forces not been watching. They swept in, arrested all six men and were led back to the apartment of a seventh, where a capsule containing the promised uranium was hidden.

By that evening, the case—the first officially acknowledged theft in Russia of weapons-grade uranium—was getting big play on local TV. The Russian police had reason to be proud; the rest of the world had one more reason to be nervous.

For while the bust was disturbing, it was hardly unique. After 60 years of building nuclear bombs and nuclear reactors, the world is fairly awash in radioactive slag—from spent fuel rods to medical waste and contaminated tools—much of it held under little if any security in labs, hospitals and factories. Even the high-test weapons-grade material that's supposed to be locked down at military installations is not as secure as it ought to be. Some weapons-storage facilities don't even have video monitors.

That such deadly material is so loosely guarded has been the source of much anxiety since [the September 11, 2001, terrorist attacks]—most of it focused on [terrorist] Osama bin Laden and [his organization] al-Qaeda. [In December 2001] reports surfaced of a meeting in Afghanistan at which an al-Qaeda associate waved a canister of what he said was nuclear material in the air to demonstrate to bin Laden and others how much progress had been made in securing the stuff.

The world is fairly awash in radioactive slag.

But bin Laden is only a part of the nuclear terror problem. Since the fall of the Soviet Union and the rise of global terrorist groups, a new market has emerged to manage the increased supply of—and demand for—nuclear contraband. More and more radioactive material has been getting filched, bundled and sent flowing through an increasingly busy pipeline from Russia and the old Soviet states into the hands, it is feared, of people desperate enough to use it.

The Russian government alone lists up to 200 terrorist organizations it believes may be trying to obtain nuclear material. In Istanbul [in November 2001], Turkish undercover officers arrested two smugglers who attempted to sell them more than 2.5 lbs. of non-weapons grade uranium for $750,000. In July [2001] police in Paris raided an apartment in which three men were holding a small quantity of highly enriched uranium and plane tickets to various East European countries.

And these busts are only the high-profile ones. Russia has broken up 601 attempted transactions since 1998. The International Atomic Energy Agency in Vienna reports 376 since 1993, and Turkey has recorded 104 cases of non-weapons grade smuggling in that same time. Moreover, for every trafficker who has been caught, chances are that many more are still in the game—a fact that has security planners deeply worried. "The global effort to control nuclear weapons is based on control of nuclear material," says Matthew Bunn, a nuclear expert at Harvard's Kennedy School of Government and a former adviser to President Bill Clinton. "If that stuff gets on the market, nothing else we do will work."

The likeliest source of most radioactive booty is Russia and the surrounding states, and the material they have to offer comes in two varieties. Top-quality, weapons-grade material is the only kind that can be used to build a true nuclear-fission bomb, and is both hard to obtain and harder to turn into an explosive. But lower-grade radioactive rubbish is also dangerous. It can be fashioned into a so-called dirty bomb: a conventional explosive packed with waste that spreads radiation in all directions.

There are at least 100 facilities around the former Soviet Union that store warheads and weapons-grade material, and most of them are reportedly not properly secured. Along the country's eastern coast, according to some sources, up to 80 abandoned, loosely guarded nuclear submarines are rusting in bays and inlets, their torpedo tubes and other openings providing possible access for intruders and an exit for radioactive leakage.

The country's nuclear power plants may be just as porous. At the Leningrad facility near the Gulf of Finland, sources say vodka and drugs flow freely among the workers, most of whom earn barely 3,000 rubles a month—about $100. Poorly paid, highly inebriated men make a shabby line of defense against terrorists and traffickers. Vaclav Havlik, a Czech citizen who was part of a group of uranium smugglers arrested near Munich in 1994, told *Time* that obtaining material from Russia was no great chore. "It was like going for vacation by the sea and bringing back a sack of shells," he says.

At the same time that smugglers are getting better at obtaining their merchandise, they are also getting smarter about transporting it. The first nuclear black marketeers carried their contraband straight out of Russia and into Europe, across some of the best-guarded borders in the world. As customs officials caught wise, the smugglers started shifting their route south, running a flanking pattern through Central Asia, the Caucasus Mountains and Turkey before resurfacing in Europe. This modified buttonhook play allows traffickers to take advantage of established drug routes—a smart strategy, since customs agents in a place such as Tajikistan, where 200 tons of drugs may cross the border on a busy day, can easily overlook a few ounces of nuclear contraband.

The black marketeers who get caught are often carrying only a few spoonfuls of nuclear material, but that's little comfort. More and more, risk-averse traffickers travel with just a taste of what they're selling rather than the entire inventory. Once they find a buyer, they can attempt the riskier business of delivering the full supply.

Just how little they would need to deliver is another source of worry. While a full-scale nuclear bomb may require 100 lbs. of enriched uranium, a more modest device, particularly one fueled by plutonium, could be built with just 10 lbs. (about 4 kg). "Four kilos of plutonium," says Lidia Popova of Russia's Center for Nuclear Ecology and Energy Policy, "is the amount that could sit in your palm."

The likeliest source of most radioactive booty is Russia and the surrounding states.

For terrorists who can't get their hands on any weapons-grade uranium, there's the option of the dirty bomb. Allied forces overrunning a suspected al-Qaeda camp in Afghanistan [in December 2001] found at least one diagram suggesting the design of such a weapon. To build this type of explosive, terrorists could use almost any kind of nuclear rubbish—perhaps even the water in Russia's Lake Karachai, a nuclear dumping ground that fairly crackles with radioactivity.

The International Atomic Energy Agency believes that dirty bombs may not be as lethal as many people assume. The explosion would be a conventional one, and the radiation might not pack much toxic wallop—depending on wind, topography and the radioactive material. The disruption, terror and economic impact, however, would be incalculable. Says Popova: "If such a bomb explodes in a city, very quickly panic will spread."

Despite all this, antiterrorism forces have reason for hope. Turkey, with the help of the U.S., has instituted stepped-up security measures at its borders, installing radiation detectors at key crossings—particularly those leading from Iraq, Iran and Georgia. (Unconfirmed reports suggest that Iran and Georgia are doing the same.) The Turkish government won't say explicitly if its security efforts have been ratcheted up since Sept. 11. "The answer is pretty obvious," says Erdener Birol, acting head of Turkey's atomic-energy authority.

To build [a dirty bomb], terrorists could use almost any kind of nuclear rubbish.

Like so much else in the terror wars however, the job of truly securing the nukes—especially in Russia—may fall to the U.S. But Washington doesn't seem to be giving the problem top priority. When the Bush Administration took office, a program was already in place to help Russia dispose of 34 tons of surplus plutonium. When the program crossed the new President's [George W. Bush] desk, however, he slashed its projected $87 million price tag, seeking just $57 million.

Washington and Moscow have also been hard at work in recent years improving security at Russia's nuclear-material storage sites, only 40% of which come up to U.S. standards. The Clinton Administration anticipated $225 million for the project [in 2001], a 30% boost over the previous year. President Bush countered with a $30 million cut. Congress kept the funding at [the 2000] level.

Perhaps the most troubled of the existing antinuclear programs is one that relies on the power of capitalism. In 1993 the U.S. agreed to buy 500 metric tons of Russian nuclear material over 20 years, blending it down to a less potent form that could be used in American nuclear power plants. So far, 137 metric tons have been processed and carried off; they account for half the nuclear fuel used in the U.S.

In 1998, however, the U.S. group authorized to buy the material was privatized. With the global market for nuclear fuel faltering, the newly profit-driven group found itself locked into the price Washington had agreed to in 1996. In an attempt to square things, the company is seeking a new contract with Russia that would guarantee it rates far below market, though talks . . . in Moscow failed to resolve the matter. If the Russians—sellers with but a single major buyer—are told they have to go along with the price cuts, the program could collapse.

For now, Washington is simply feeling its way, trying to balance security and cost while tending to the countless other battles it must fight on the home front. Given the power of even a single rogue nuke, however, this battle is clearly one of the most important. "The consequences of failure would be far worse than Sept. 11," says Alexander Strezov, a Bulgarian scientist who helps investigate trafficking cases. "To be honest, I don't want to think about it." The U.S., unfortunately, doesn't have that luxury.

4

Terrorists Are Unlikely to Use Nuclear Weapons

Gary Milhollin

Gary Milhollin directs the Wisconsin Project on Nuclear Arms Control in Washington, D.C.

Terrorists seeking nuclear weapons would either have to build them from scratch or procure them on the black market, both extremely difficult feats. Building a nuclear bomb from scratch would require making bomb-grade fuel. However, manufacturing such radioactive material would require a tremendous amount of equipment, which would be nearly impossible to purchase and conceal. Buying fuel would entail the same problems as trying to buy ready-to-use nuclear weapons: Most nations are unlikely to sell such items to terrorist groups. Even if terrorists were able to procure enough radioactive material to build conventional bombs that would disperse radiation when exploded, any such bomb radioactive enough to cause widespread harm would be too dangerous for terrorists to handle.

The story began over a meal in late October [2001]. [A] high British official told a reporter from the *London Times* that [terrorist] Osama bin Laden had the bomb, or at least that he had gotten bomb components, or nuclear materials, and that the source was Pakistan. At about the same time, Pakistan arrested three of its nuclear scientists for questioning about possible ties to the Taliban, bin Laden's Afghan protectors. Then, in early November, bin Laden himself declared that he had nuclear weapons, which he would use as a "deterrent."

A lower risk than most people think

Could it be true? Countries do not arrest their nuclear scientists for nothing. By mid-November, Graham Allison, a professor at Harvard and an assistant secretary of defense in the Clinton administration, was predicting in the *Washington Post* that "bin Laden's final act could be a nuclear at-

Gary Milhollin, "Can Terrorists Get the Bomb?" *Commentary*, vol. 113, February 2002, pp. 45–50.

tack on America." A few weeks later, the *Post*'s Bob Woodward reported that [bin Laden's organization] al Qaeda might be making a "dirty" bomb—a radiological device to spread contamination over a wide area. According to Woodward, this could be done by wrapping spent reactor fuel rods around high explosives, which would produce a "zone of intense radiation that could extend several city blocks." A larger bomb, he said, "could affect a much larger area."

In Afghanistan itself, American forces have examined dozens of sites where al Qaeda may have worked on nuclear or radiological weapons. Secretary of Defense Donald Rumsfeld cautioned that while it was "unlikely that they have a nuclear weapon," considering "the determination they have, they may very well."

Despite the reports, and despite the attendant warnings, the risk that a terrorist group like al Qaeda could get the bomb (or a "dirty" substitute) is much lower than most people think. That is the good news. There is also bad news: the risk is not zero.

Building from scratch

There are essentially two ways for a terrorist group to lay its hands on a nuclear weapon: either build one from scratch or somehow procure an already manufactured one or its key components. Neither of these is likely.

Building a bomb from scratch would confer the most power: a group that could build one bomb could build several, and a nuclear arsenal would put it front and center on the world stage. But of all the possibilities, this is the unlikeliest—"so remote,"—in the words of a senior nuclear scientist at the Los Alamos National Laboratory, "that it can be essentially ruled out." The chief obstacle lies in producing the nuclear fuel—either bomb-grade uranium or plutonium—that actually explodes in a chain reaction. More than 80 percent of the effort that went into making America's first bombs was devoted to producing this fuel, and it is no easy task.

The chief obstacle [to building a nuclear bomb] lies in producing the nuclear fuel.

To make bomb-grade uranium, a terrorist group would need thousands of high-speed gas centrifuges, machined to exact dimensions, arranged in series, and capable of operating under the most demanding conditions. If they wanted to produce the uranium by a diffusion process, they would need an even greater number of other machines, equally difficult to manufacture and operate. If they followed [former Iraqi leader] Saddam Hussein's example, they could try building a series of giant electromagnets, capable of bending a stream of electrically charged particles—a no less daunting challenge. For any of these, they would also need a steady supply of natural uranium and a specialized plant to convert it to a gaseous form for processing.

Who would sell these things to would-be nuclear terrorists? The answer is: nobody. The world's nuclear-equipment makers are organized into a cooperative group that exists precisely to stop items like these from getting into unauthorized hands. Nor could a buyer disguise the destination and send materials through obliging places like Dubai (as Iran does with its hot cargoes) or Malta (favored by Libya's smugglers). The equipment is so specialized, and the suppliers so few, that a forest of red flags would go up. And even if the equipment could be bought, it would have to be operated in a place that the United States could not find.

Plutonium is only created inside reactor fuel rods, and the rods . . . become so hot that they melt unless kept under water.

If manufacturing bomb-grade uranium is out of the picture, what about making plutonium, a much smaller quantity of which is required to form a critical mass (less than fourteen pounds was needed to destroy Nagasaki in 1945)? There is, however, an inconvenient fact about plutonium, which is that you need a reactor to make enough of it for a workable bomb. Could terrorists buy one? The Russians are selling a reactor to Iran, but Moscow tends to put terrorist groups in the same category as Chechens [dissidents from Chechnya it considers terrorists]. The Chinese are selling reactors to Pakistan, but Beijing, too, is not fond of terrorists. India and Pakistan can both build reactors on their own, but, for now, these countries are lined up with the U.S. Finally, smuggling a reactor would be no easier than buying one. Reactor parts are unique, so manufacturers would not be fooled by phony purchase orders.

Even if terrorists somehow got hold of a reactor, they would need a special, shielded chemical plant to chop up its radioactive fuel, dissolve it in acid, and then extract the plutonium from the acid. No one would sell them a plutonium extraction plant, either.

It is worth remembering that Saddam Hussein tried the reactor road in the 1970's. He bought one from France—[French president] Jacques Chirac, in his younger days, was a key facilitator of the deal—hoping it would propel Iraq into the nuclear club. But the reactor's fuel was sabotaged in a French warehouse, the person who was supposed to certify its quality was murdered in a Paris hotel, and when the reactor was finally ready to operate, a squadron of Israeli fighter-bombers blew it apart. A similar fate would undoubtedly await any group that tried to follow Saddam's method today.

Procuring nuclear fuel

If making nuclear-bomb fuel is a no-go, why not just steal it, or buy it on the black market? Consider plutonium. There are hundreds of reactors in the world, and they crank out tons of the stuff every year. Surely a dedicated band of terrorists could get their hands on some.

This too is not so simple. Plutonium is only created inside reactor fuel rods, and the rods, after being irradiated, become so hot that they melt unless kept under water. They are also radioactive, which is why they have to travel submerged from the reactor to storage ponds, with the water acting as both coolant and radiation shield. And in most power reactors, the rods are welded together into long assemblies that can be lifted only by crane.

True, after the rods cool down they can be stored dry, but their radioactivity is still lethal. To prevent spent fuel rods from killing the people who come near them, they are transported in giant radiation-shielding casks that are not supposed to break open even in head-on collisions. The casks are also guarded. If terrorists managed to hijack one from a country that had reactors they would still have to take it to a plant in another country that could extract the plutonium from the rods. They would be hunted at every step of the way.

Instead of fuel rods, they would be better advised to go after pure plutonium, already removed from the reactor fuel and infinitely easier to handle. This kind of plutonium is a threat only if you ingest or inhale it. Human skin blocks its radiation: a terrorist could walk around with a lump of it in his front trouser pocket and still have children. But where to get hold of it? Russia is the best bet: it has tons of plutonium in weapon-ready form, and the Russian nuclear-accounting system is weak. Russia also has underpaid scientists, and there is unquestionably some truth behind all the stories one hears about the smuggling that goes on in that country.

The problem with buying bomb-grade uranium is that one would need a great deal of it.

But very little Russian plutonium has been in circulation, with not a single reported case of anything more than gram quantities showing up on the black market. This makes sense. Pure plutonium is used primarily for making nuclear warheads, it is in military hands, and military forces are not exactly keen to see it come back at them in somebody else's bombs.

One source of pure plutonium that is not military is a new kind of reactor fuel called "mixed oxide." It is very different from the present generation of fuel because it contains weapon-ready material. But precisely because it is weapon-ready, it is guarded and accounted for, and a terrorist group would have to win a gun battle to get close to it. Then they would probably need a crane to move it, and would have to elude or fight off their pursuers.

If terrorists did procure some weapon-ready plutonium, would their problems be over? Far from it: plutonium works only in an "implosion"-type bomb, which is about ten times more difficult to build than the simple uranium bomb used at Hiroshima [during World War II]. In such a device, a spherical shock wave "implodes" inward and squeezes a ball of plutonium at the bomb's center so that it explodes in a chain reaction. To accomplish all this, one needs precision machine tools to build the parts, special furnaces to melt and cast the plutonium in a vacuum (liquid plutonium oxidizes rapidly in air), and high-precision switches and capacitors for the firing circuit. Also required are a qualified designer, a number of other specialists, and a testing program. Considering who the participating scientists are likely to be, the chances of getting an implosion bomb to work are rather small.

Bomb-grade uranium

The alternative to plutonium is bomb-grade uranium—and here things would be easier. This is the fuel used in the Hiroshima bomb. Unlike the implosion bomb dropped on Nagasaki, this one did not have to be tested: the U.S. knew it would work. The South Africans built six uranium bombs without testing; they knew their bombs would work, too. All these devices used a simple "gun" design in which one slug of uranium was shot down a barrel into another.

The problem with buying bomb-grade uranium is that one would need a great deal of it—around 120 pounds for a gun-type bomb—and nothing near that amount has turned up in the black market. In February 2001 an al Qaeda operative named Jamal Ahmed al-Fadl testified in an American court that he had tried to buy some uranium for $1.5 million in 1993. He had been sent to Khartoum, where he saw a cylinder that supposedly contained uranium from South Africa; he did not know whether the deal went through. South Africa went out of the nuclear-weapon business in 1991, and in 1993 it accounted for all of its bomb-grade uranium to the International Atomic Energy Agency. The deal in Khartoum was probably a scam.

What about getting material from Pakistan? Its centrifuges have been turning out bomb-grade uranium since 1986, and by now there is enough for 30 to 50 nuclear weapons. As is well known, at least some of its nuclear scientists have fundamentalist leanings. Could they spirit out enough for a bomb or two?

The chances are virtually nil. Pakistan's nuclear weapons are its proudest achievement. Every gram of bomb-grade uranium has been produced at the expense of the country's suffering population, and every gram is also part of a continuous manufacturing flow. When uranium leaves the centrifuges, it goes to other plants where it is refined and then to still other plants where it is made into bombs. Pakistan produces enough for about three bombs per year, which means that one bomb's worth is the result of several months' output.

> *[Terrorists] would have to design the bomb, develop it, and build it, and that would be far from a trivial undertaking.*

If any uranium went missing, it would be as if the assembly workers for Ford Explorers suddenly stopped receiving engines. Someone down the production line would be bound to ask questions, and very quickly.

There is also the fact that Pakistan's nuclear program is controlled by the army, still headed by the country's president, Pervez Musharraf. In response to the September 11 [2001] terrorist attack on America, Musharraf created a new military command with direct control over the nuclear-weapons program. In the process, he sidelined officers sympathetic to the Taliban. After all these precautions, Musharraf is unlikely to let any bomb fuel slip through his fingers. The only possibility for terrorists to lay their hands on Pakistan's uranium would be if its government fell under the control of sympathizers; given that Pakistan's army is far and away the most effective and stable organization in the country, there is not much chance of that.

Russia, again, is the best bet. It has tons of bomb-grade uranium left over from the cold war and, in addition to bombs, has used this material to fuel nuclear submarines and research reactors. The result has been to spread it across Russia and several other former members of the eastern bloc.

A bomb that carried enough radiation to injure many people quickly would be too hot to handle.

So Russia and its former satellites are a fat target. This past November [2001], citing a database maintained by the International Atomic Energy Agency, the *New York Times* catalogued a long series of Russian-related smuggling attempts. In 1993, for example, over six pounds of weapon-grade uranium in St. Petersburg was about to go astray before being seized; in 1998, there was a foiled effort to steal more than 40 pounds in the Urals. Russian officials told the *Times* that they had twice discovered terrorists staking out their nuclear-weapon sites. Finally, there was one loss "of the highest consequence" during the past year, about which details were not forthcoming.

Building and getting caught

There are thus definite prospects in Russia. If terrorists could strike the mother lode, and get enough uranium for a gun-type bomb, they would be on their way.

But the way would still be long. They would have to design the bomb, develop it, and build it, and that would be far from a trivial undertaking. They would have to have a competent bomb designer, who could be a physicist or engineer but would have to come with practical experience in making such things work. High-accuracy machine tools could be dispensed with—implosion not being required, much simpler technologies could be used for firing projectiles down artillery tubes—although someone would have to handle the uranium-235, refine it to metallic form, cast it, and then machine it. Still, with the help of a capable machinist and a chemical laboratory, none of these obstacles is insurmountable.

The main risk would lie in getting caught. True, a uranium bomb would not produce many of the "signatures" that American intelligence agencies look for—the use of a lot of electricity (a sign of uranium enrichment plant), the presence of contaminated air or water (a sign of a reactor or plutonium extraction plant), a noisy testing program—but a fair number of people would have to be recruited, and one of them could turn the others in. Purchase of equipment might arouse the suspicions of a seller. Above all, what would be needed is a sanctuary—a place in which to assemble the people and the equipment, and keep them together for a period of time. You cannot transport such an operation from cave to cave.

Finding this location would not be easy. A country that was aware of the terrorists' program could end up getting blamed for a nuclear attack on America, and not too many governments would be ready to sign up for that. Better from the terrorists' viewpoint would be a location where the authorities had no idea what they were doing, but even so the theft of the uranium would probably be discovered soon enough, and it might be only a short matter of time before the whole world showed up on their doorstep. Besides, if they only managed to steal enough for one bomb, they would still lack an arsenal—and a single mistake in design could wreck the whole project.

Is there no way around these manufacturing problems? There is: stealing, or buying, a complete bomb. But this presents problems of its own, which are even greater.

The job of making or procuring a nuclear bomb is a great deal harder than we have been led to believe.

All countries, including Russia and Pakistan, take care to safeguard their warheads, and even rogue states, if they should get the bomb, would be highly likely to do the same. Despite press speculation to the contrary, countries maintain careful inventories and employ security measures specifically designed to prevent theft. Warheads are typically stored in bunkers to which access is tightly restricted. They are also protected by alarms and armed guards. Terrorists would have a hard fight on their hands taking over one of these bunkers, and even if they succeeded, they would have a much harder fight getting away with the contents.

Buying is not a great option, either. Since the 1970's, the Libyan dictator Muammar Qaddafi has tried to buy nuclear weapons from China, India, and Pakistan, reportedly offering billions of dollars. So far, there have been no takers. In 1996, General Alexander Lebed, then vying for the presidency of Russia, claimed that a number of "suitcase" bombs—meant to be carried by foot soldiers on demolition missions—had gone missing, but his claim was promptly denied by both the Russian and U.S. governments and has never gained much credibility. In November 2001, [Russian] President Vladimir Putin said he could certify that no Russian warheads had fallen into terrorist hands.

Dirty bombs

What options remain? Stymied in their plan to acquire a real nuclear weapon, could a determined group of terrorists at least confirm Bob Woodward's fears by manufacturing a "dirty" bomb? Such a device would be much easier to build than a warhead. Instead of producing a nuclear explosion, it would only have to disperse radioactive particles.

This is a likelier bet. But there is a different problem with these devices: they do not pack much radioactive punch. A bomb that carried enough radiation to injure many people quickly would be too hot to handle. The shielding would have to be many times heavier than the radioactive element—so massive, in fact, that there would be no practical way to transport or deploy the weapon. That is why the Pentagon does not consider such devices useful on the battlefield.

Nor is it easy to bring a sufficient amount of radioactivity into contact with a bomb's human targets. Lacing a high-explosive charge with nuclear waste from a hospital or laboratory, for example, would kill some people immediately from the explosion, but the only radiological effect would be an increased risk of cancer decades later. Once the area around the blast was decontaminated, it would be safer to walk through it than to be a serious smoker.

To inflict a dangerous dose over a broad area requires spewing around large amounts of nuclear waste. The only place to get such waste would be from a reactor, and the problems with that scenario have already been demonstrated. Even if a group of terrorists could somehow procure radioactive fuel rods or any other form of highly radioactive waste, wrapping the rods around "readily available conventional high explosives," as Woodward suggested in the *Post*, would kill the person doing the wrapping. So would transporting such a weapon to its destination, unless the rods were heavily shielded during the entire operation (which would bring us back to the implausible scenario with the giant protective casks). The fact is that it would be a near impossibility to create, in Woodward's words, a "zone of intense radiation that could extend several city blocks."

A research reactor would be a better source. Many countries use such small reactors to irradiate material samples, and it might be possible to insert some material into one of these reactors secretly, irradiate it, and then withdraw it and put it in a bomb. The difficulty would then lie in making the bomb effective. Highly radioactive materials have short half-lives; thus, any bomb would have to be used right away, and one would not be able to build up a stockpile. If enough radioactivity were packed into the bomb to injure a substantial number of victims, the too-hot-to-handle problem would arise. If the radioactive charge were diluted, the bomb would lose its effect. Saddam Hussein actually made and tested such a bomb in the 1980's, but when UN inspectors toured the test site in the 1990's they could find no trace of radiation from it.

Other uses of nuclear material

What about putting plutonium into a city's drinking water, or into the air? That, too, is a possibility—but according to a 1995 study by the Lawrence Livermore National Laboratory, plutonium dumped into a typical city reservoir would almost entirely sink to the bottom. The little that dissolved would be greatly diluted by the volume of the water, and the people drinking it would get a smaller dose than from natural background radiation. As for plutonium in the air, if an entire kilogram of the stuff were exploded in a city the size of Munich, Germany, and if 20 percent of it became airborne in respirable particles—as with anthrax, the particles would have to be the right size to lodge in the lungs—the effect (according to the same study) would be to produce fewer than ten deaths from cancer.

The main effect of any of these attacks would be panic: people would flee the contaminated zone. This might create a huge economic impact—which would be a victory for the terrorists—and it would be almost certain to create an even huger psychological impact. On the other hand, and unlike anthrax, radiation is something that scientists know how to detect, and at levels far below those that are dangerous. Even the panic might fade quickly as people were reassured that the environment was safe. In any case, there is no chance of achieving anything remotely like the effect of a real nuclear weapon, however small.

Preventing ground zero

In sum, the job of making or procuring a nuclear bomb is a great deal harder than we have been led to believe. From a terrorist's point of view, what is clear above all is that, whether the aim is to build a dirty bomb or a clean one, a sanctuary is needed. The task requires laboratories, equipment, and trained personnel, all of which have to be maintained over a longish period of time.

This in turn underlines the cardinal importance of remaining faithful to our determination to pursue terrorists everywhere, and never leave them in peace. Allowing any group of terrorists to set up shop anywhere puts everyone at risk.

The terrorists' only hope is that we tire of the chase. Then, if they could obtain the bomb, they could deliver it, and anywhere on the globe could become ground zero.

5

Iran Poses a Serious Threat to Nuclear Security

Leonard S. Spector

Leonard S. Spector is deputy director of the Monterey Institute Center for Nonproliferation Studies and leads its Washington, D.C., office.

Iran has made progress in developing nuclear weapons despite international efforts to stop it. At the end of 2002, UN inspectors discovered that Iran had built a facility to enrich uranium, which is used to make nuclear bombs. The nation had also erected a plant to produce heavy water, which is used in reactors to produce plutonium, another weapons fuel. Since international monitoring and nonproliferation controls have failed to curtail Iran's nuclear ambitions, the international community must isolate Iran until it complies with international nonproliferation laws.

As the [George W.] Bush Administration took office in January 2001, Iran presented a classic nuclear proliferation challenge that appeared to be manageable with traditional nonproliferation tools. Today, however, the U.S. believes the challenge is far more serious than previously thought, and that the tools for addressing it are no longer sufficient. At the upcoming June [2003] meeting of the UN's International Atomic Energy Agency (IAEA), Washington wants the agency to declare Iran in material breach of its nonproliferation obligations. The Bush Administration fears that the development of an Iranian bomb—a project which now appears to have been bolstered by clandestine foreign assistance—could have far-reaching consequences.

The seeming success of nonproliferation tools

For the past decade, Iran has been trying to complete a nuclear power reactor at Bushehr, begun with German assistance during the time of the Shah. Germany froze further cooperation after the 1979 Iranian Revolution. After a period of opposing all programs symbolizing modernization, Iran's Islamic revolutionary leaders signed an agreement with Russia to complete the facility. Tehran has never offered a convincing justification for why it needs the facility, given the fact that it could much more quickly and cheaply use its natural gas resources (much of it flared off) to fuel any needed electricity production. U.S. observers have seen it as a cover to permit the development of more sensitive nuclear facilities that could support a nuclear weapons program.

In early 2001, it was assumed that Iran was seeking to acquire nuclear arms, but there was little evidence that it was progressing. Washington had succeeded in persuading Russia to hold up the export of lasers that might have been usable for enriching uranium from its natural state to weapons-grade. (It takes about 25 kg of enriched uranium to make a Hiroshima style bomb.) While the Bush Administration, like its predecessor, believed Iran was pursuing other options to develop the bomb, there was also little evidence that it was succeeding. Since 1991, when Iraq was found to have clandestinely developed nuclear facilities despite its adherence to the Non-Proliferation Treaty (NPT), the UN's International Atomic Energy Agency (IAEA) asserted the right to demand a special inspection of a suspect undeclared site in an NPT-party state. In 2001, it appeared that this reinforced international inspection system could be used to keep Iran on the defensive. At the first indication from U.S. intelligence that Iran was building a clandestine nuclear facility, the IAEA could demand a look, and international pressure would build for Iran to halt the apparent violation of its nonproliferation pledges.

Export controls by industrialized nations were a second arrow in the quiver of nonproliferation tools. As the result of concerted U.S. diplomacy in the 1980s, China had ceased nuclear cooperation with Iran, a nuclear embargo by Western nuclear suppliers was holding firm, and, through constant U.S. intervention, it was hoped that leakage of sensitive nuclear technology from Russia could be halted.

The discovery of Iran's nuclear progress

By the end of 2002, this hopeful view of the international nonproliferation regime was dashed by the discovery that in the previous 18–24 months, despite the vigilance of U.S. and other intelligence services, Iran had secretly made considerable progress on two different routes to nuclear weapons.

Iran had secretly made considerable progress on two different routes to nuclear weapons.

First, it had completed a pilot-scale facility to enrich uranium at Natanz using high-speed centrifuges, a demanding technology but one that is now spreading rapidly. If enlarged, the facility would be capable of producing large quantities of uranium enriched to the level needed for nuclear weapons of the type used against Hiroshima [during World War II]. Second, Iran appeared to have completed, or to be near completing, a facility at Arak for the production of heavy water, a product used in reactors designed to produce plutonium. This was the material used in the

Nagasaki bomb [during World War II].

The advanced state of these facilities was doubly disturbing because it implied that Iran possessed still other, as yet undeclared nuclear plants. When the IAEA's Director-General, Mohammed El Baradei, eventually requested and was granted a visit to the Natanz facility, his team concluded that the facility was so sophisticated that it could only have been built after Iran had constructed and operated a smaller scale, experimental enrichment unit. While Iran might claim that it had no obligation to declare the Natanz plant because it had not yet introduced natural uranium into the facility, it would have had to take this step to test out the smaller experimental facility—a clear violation of its inspection obligations under the NPT.

Iran will now merely go through the motions of complying with the [UN's monitoring] system, while continuing to pursue clandestine nuclear activities.

Moreover, the fact that Iran was attempting to produce heavy water implied that it was constructing—or had completed—a heavy-water-using reactor, which it had also not declared. (Heavy water is not needed for the nuclear power plant that Russia is building for Iran, at Bushehr.)

Monitoring and export controls proved ineffective

Thus, far from keeping Iran off balance and on the defensive, IAEA monitoring had apparently missed at least two, and possibly four, sensitive installations.

Export controls, obviously, had proven no more effective. It is highly unlikely that Iran developed uranium enrichment centrifuge technology on its own, although who may have assisted Iran to obtain it remains unclear. North Korea is one possibility. It is believed to have traded medium-range No-Dong missiles to Pakistan in return for centrifuge enrichment know-how and, possibly, centrifuge prototypes. At the time, North Korea was also selling the No-Dong to Iran, for cash. It is not unreasonable to imagine Pyongyang struck a second bargain with Tehran to sell it Pakistani-origin enrichment technology.

It is also possible that Pakistan might have made the sale directly. Elements of Pakistan's leadership share an anti-Western, fundamentalist Islamic outlook with their Iranian counterparts, although historically, Pakistan's Sunni Muslims have not made common cause with Iran's Shias.

Still less is known about the origins of Iran's heavy water production capabilities. Iran has now declared that it will place the Natanz facility under IAEA inspection to ensure that its output is used only for non-military purposes; under existing IAEA rules Iran need not do the same for the Arak plant. But inspections will not solve the Iranian nuclear challenge.

First, the United States has declared its view that Iran has violated the inspection requirements of the NPT, in particular because of its failure to declare the predecessor facility to the Natanz plant. Given this history, Washington must now be concerned that, like Iraq, Iran will now merely go through the motions of complying with the IAEA system, while continuing to pursue clandestine nuclear activities. Indeed, during the UN debate in the run-up to the war against Iraq [in 2003], the Bush Administration declared that inspections—even those of the UN Monitoring and Verification Commission, which had far greater powers than the IAEA—could not effectively disarm a state intent on retaining weapons of mass destruction.

No less troubling is the "break-out" scenario. Under the NPT, Iran is permitted to enrich uranium, even to weapons grade, as long as the material is kept under IAEA inspection. The treaty also permits states to withdraw from it on 90 days notice, if its supreme national interests are threatened.

Thus, even if Iran complied impeccably with its IAEA obligations, over time, it could amass a stockpile of enriched uranium. Then, if at some future juncture it found itself threatened by the United States or a resurgent Iraq, it could withdraw from the NPT, seize this stockpile, and manufacture nuclear weapons in a matter of weeks. Indeed, even if it produced stocks only of low-enriched uranium of the type used in the Bushehr reactor, Iran's centrifuge enrichment plant could be rapidly modified to "re-enrich" the material and bring it to weapons grade in a few weeks' time.

International censure

What options remain for constraining Iran's nuclear ambitions? If the Bush Administration can rally the international community to condemn Iran and isolate it diplomatically, it may be able to push Iran for concessions. The first would be for Iran to accept the "Additional Protocol" to its safeguards agreement. The protocol, developed after the 1991 Gulf War, would give the IAEA de jure authority to hunt for suspect plants and to keep tabs on activities beyond the agency's usual mandate, like heavy water production. If that were coupled with Iran's agreement to freeze the Natanz and Arak facilities, without operating them, the United States and other concerned parties might breathe somewhat easier.

Unfortunately, with Iran's revolutionary faction still controlling the country's national security policy and seemingly more emboldened each day as it sees new opportunities for influence in Southern Iraq, the prospects for such a turnaround in Iran's nuclear posture appear all too distant.

6

India and Pakistan Pose a Serious Threat to Nuclear Security

Pervez Hoodbhoy

Pervez Hoodbhoy is a professor of high-energy physics at Quaid-e-Azam University in Islamabad, Pakistan. He is also a member of the Bulletin of the Atomic Scientists' *Board of Sponsors.*

Pakistan's and India's nuclear capabilities are uniquely dangerous. First, these nations actively fight over disputed territory, making a war in which nuclear weapons are used more likely. Second, unlike other nations that possess nuclear weapons, India and Pakistan seem ignorant of the devastation such weapons can cause. Last, Pakistanis and Indians are especially fearless people, believing that divine forces protect them. This ignorance and fearlessness combined with ongoing war over Kashmir could lead to a nuclear catastrophe in Southeast Asia.

For more than a decade before India initiated nuclear testing in May 1998, the rival nuclear tribes in Pakistan and India had pleaded for converting their respective country's covert nuclear program into an overt one. They argued that because war between two nuclear states was impossible, unsheathing the bomb would bring an era of unprecedented peace, stability, and reduced defense budgets.

They could not have been more wrong. Since January [2002], thousands of artillery shells have been exchanged across the Line of Control in Kashmir [a disputed territory], destroying the lives of border residents. By May, a million troops glowered at each other across the border; some Indian and Pakistani cities tested their air raid sirens. On into June, as tensions mounted, world leaders worked overtime to prevent tensions between Pakistan and India from exploding into war.

As of August, although troops have not yet been demobilized, tempers are down a notch, and a semblance of normalcy has emerged. But even at the peak of the crisis, few Indians or Pakistanis lost much sleep.

Pervez Hoodbhoy, "Nuclear Gamblers: We Can Make a First Strike, and a Second, or Even a Third," *Bulletin of the Atomic Scientists*, vol. 58, September/October 2002, p. 26. Copyright © 2002 by the Educational Foundation for Nuclear Science, Inc. Reproduced by permission.

Stock markets flickered, but there was no run on the banks or panic buying. Schools and colleges, which generally close at the first hint of crisis, functioned normally.

A fierce and suicidal struggle

The outside world saw the situation in very different terms—as a fierce and suicidal struggle between two nuclear-armed states. But while foreign nationals streamed out of both countries, we saw the crisis as more of the usual—except that the rhetoric was a bit fiercer and the saber-rattling a bit louder.

In a public debate in Islamabad [Pakistan], Gen. Mirza Aslam Beg, the former chief of Pakistan's army, declared: "We can make a first strike, and a second strike, or even a third."

The lethality of nuclear war left him unmoved. "You can die crossing the street," he observed, "or you could die in a nuclear war. You've got to die some day anyway."

Across the border, India's Defence Minister George Fernandes, in an interview with the *Hindustan Times*, voiced similar sentiments: "We could take a strike, survive, and then hit back. Pakistan would be finished." Indian Defence Secretary Yogendra Narain took things a step further in an interview with *Outlook Magazine:* "A surgical strike is the answer." But, he added, if that failed to resolve things, "We must be prepared for total mutual destruction." A hawkish Indian security analyst, Brahma Chellaney, demanded that India "call Pakistan's nuclear bluff."

Pakistan and India are making history in their own way. No other nuclear states have engaged in such fiery rhetoric, no matter how great the tension between them. The fear of mutual destruction has always put sharp limits on the tone and volume of nuclear rhetoric. So, what accounts for the extraordinary difference between us Pakistanis and Indians and the rest of the world? What makes us such extraordinarily bold nuclear gamblers, playing close to the brink?

> *No other nuclear states have engaged in such fiery rhetoric, no matter how great the tension between them.*

In part, the answer has to do with the fact that India and Pakistan are societies in which the fundamental belief structure demands disempowerment and surrender to larger forces. A fatalistic Hindu belief that the stars above determine our destiny, and the equivalent Muslim belief in qismet, certainly account for part of it. Conversations and discussions often end with the remark that "what will be, will be," after which people shrug their shoulders and move on to something else. Because they feel they will be protected by larger, unseen forces, the level of risk-taking is extraordinary. (Any trip on the madly careening public buses in either Karachi or Bombay—which routinely smash into and kill pedestrians—proves the point.)

But other reasons may be more important.

Close government control over national television, especially in Pakistan, has ensured that critical discussion of nuclear weapons and nuclear war is not aired. Instead, in Pakistan's public squares and at crossroads stand missiles and fiberglass replicas of the nuclear test site. For the masses, they are symbols of national glory and achievement, not of death and destruction.

Nuclear ignorance is the norm

Nuclear ignorance is the norm, extending even to the educated. When asked, some students at the university in Islamabad where I teach said that a nuclear war would be the end of the world. Others thought nukes were just bigger bombs. Many said it was the army's concern, not theirs. Almost none knew about the possibility of a nuclear firestorm, residual radioactivity, or damage to the gene pool.

Because nuclear war is considered a distant abstraction, civil defense in both countries is nonexistent. As India's Adm. Ramu Ramdas, now retired and a leading peace activist, caustically remarked, "There are no air raid shelters in this city of Delhi, because in this country people are considered expendable."

Ignorance and its attendant lack of fear make it easier for [Pakistani and Indian] leaders to treat their people as pawns in a mad nuclear game.

Islamabad's civil defense budget is a laughable $40,000 and the current year's [2002] allocation has yet to be disbursed. No serious contingency plans have been devised—plans that might save millions of lives by providing timely information about escape routes, sources of nonradioactive food and drinking water, or iodine tablets.

Ignorance and its attendant lack of fear make it easier for leaders to treat their people as pawns in a mad nuclear game. How else to explain Indian Prime Minister Atal Bihari Vajpayee's recent exhortations to his troops in Kashmir to prepare for "decisive victory"? His nuclear brinksmanship is made possible by influential Indian experts seeking to trivialize Pakistan's nuclear capability. Such analysts have gained wide currency, offering instant security to all who choose to believe them.

The reasoning of the "trivialization school" goes as follows: Pakistan is a client state of the United States, and Pakistani nuclear weapons are under U.S. control. In an extreme crisis, the United States would either prohibit their use or, if need be, destroy them.

At a January [2002] meeting in Dubai, senior Indian analysts said they were "bored" with Pakistan's nuclear threats and no longer believed them. K. Subrahmanyam, an influential hawk who has advocated overt Indian nuclearization for more than a decade, believes that India can "sleep in peace."

Indian denial of Pakistani capabilities is not a new phenomenon. Two months before the May 1998 nuclear tests by India and Pakistan, a delegation from Pugwash, an international organization of scientists concerned about nuclear war, met in Delhi with Prime Minister Inder Kumar Gujral. A member of the delegation, I expressed worries about a nuclear catastrophe on the Subcontinent. Gujral repeatedly assured me—both in public and in private—that Pakistan was not capable of making atomic bombs.

He was not alone. Senior Indian defense analysts like P.R. Chari had also published articles before May 1998 arguing this point, as had the former head of the Indian Atomic Energy Agency, Dr. Raja Ramana.

Pakistan proved the doubters wrong. Forced out of the closet by the Indian tests, Pakistan's nuclear weapons gave the country a false sense of confidence and security. This encouraged it to launch its secret war in the Kargil area of Kashmir. India wanted to respond, but the existence of Pakistan's deterrence sharply limited its options.

September 11 changed everything

Then came [the September 11, 2001, terrorist attacks on America]. In a global climate deeply hostile to Islamic militancy, new possibilities opened up to India. Seeking to settle the score, India now began to seriously consider cross-border strikes on militant camps on the Pakistani side of the Line of Control. To sell the idea to the Indian public, it became essential to deny the potency of Pakistan's nuclear weapons.

But to fearlessly challenge a nuclear Pakistan requires the denial of reality. It is an enormous leap of faith to presume that the United States would have either the intention—or the power—to destroy Pakistani nukes. Tracking and destroying even a handful of mobile nuclear-armed missiles would be no easy feat.

In 1991, U.S. efforts to destroy Iraqi Scuds had limited success. No country has ever tried to take out another's nuclear bombs. It would be fantastically dangerous because one needs 100 percent success.

Even as the current missile crisis winds down, the obvious question is: how long before the two countries end up once again on the nuclear brink? Ignorant and fearless, India and Pakistan could well add a new chapter to the well-worn textbooks on the theory of nuclear deterrence.

7

North Korea Poses a Serious Threat to Nuclear Security

Joshua Muravchik

Joshua Muravchik is a resident scholar at the American Enterprise Institute, a scholarly research institute that is dedicated to preserving limited government, private enterprise, and a strong foreign policy and national defense.

In 2002 North Korea stated that it was developing nuclear weapons despite international prohibitions against it. These actions are simply part of North Korea's ongoing history of noncooperation with international treaties, to which America consistently responds with appeasement. Over the course of twenty years, a series of U.S. presidents tried and failed to contain North Korea's nuclear ambitions. Proposed responses to the 2002 threats promise to be equally ineffective. The only way to make the world safe from North Korea is to depose its leader, Kim Jong Il, through military action.

Early last October [2002], North Korea admitted that it had been secretly continuing to develop nuclear weapons despite a 1994 agreement with the U.S. not to. The confession was unapologetic. Not only, said North Korean officials, did they have the uranium-enrichment program that the U.S. had come to suspect them of having, but they possessed other, "more powerful" things as well.

New threats from North Korea

In the period that followed, Pyongyang responded with mounting belligerence to criticism of its defiant violation of the 1994 agreement. For the first time it openly acknowledged that it actually possessed nuclear weapons (although denying it the very next day). It also began to thaw a "frozen" plutonium program, taking steps to reactivate the nuclear reactor and reprocessing facility at Yongbyon that had been shut down under the same 1994 accord, expelling the International Atomic Energy Agency

Joshua Muravchik, "Facing Up to North Korea," *Commentary*, vol. 115, March 2003, p. 33.

(IAEA) inspectors who were monitoring the site, dismantling IAEA's surveillance equipment, and apparently beginning to remove from storage the fuel rods from which bomb material is directly produced. Ratcheting tensions further, it declared its withdrawal from the nuclear non-proliferation treaty (NPT), warned Japan that it was going to renew its testing of ballistic missiles, and, for good measure, threatened the U.S. with "uncontrollable catastrophe."

Ratcheting tensions further, [North Korea] declared its withdrawal from the nuclear non-proliferation treaty.

In the face of all this, and caught in the midst of a confrontation with [Iraqi leader] Saddam Hussein,[1] the Bush administration tried hard to keep its cool. Together with South Korea and Japan, it suspended shipments of the oil that the three countries had been donating to Pyongyang under the 1994 deal; and it beefed up U.S. forces in the region somewhat. But President [George W.] Bush and his team also took pains to stress that they sought a diplomatic resolution of the crisis. Insisting at first that we would not "negotiate," the administration soon made it clear by a series of small capitulations that this was not the case, and even began to hint at some of the inducements it was prepared to offer. Playing down the gravity of the situation, Secretary of State Colin Powell asked, rhetorically, "What are they going to do with another two or three more nuclear weapons when they're starving, when they have no energy, when they have no economy that's functioning?"

Unfortunately, Powell's question answers itself. Pyongyang's first few nuclear weapons have presumably been reserved against the possibility that America might "go nuclear" in defense of South Korea, and in order to extort succor from frightened nations near and far. As for any additional weapons, what it is likely to do with them is to sell them—just as it has already sold nuclear-capable missiles to Iran, Libya, Syria, and, most recently, Yemen. Such weapons would bring a pretty penny on the well-established trade routes that connect Pyongyang to Tehran, Tripoli, and Damascus, or new ones that may reach to the murky haunts of [terrorist] Osama bin Laden and the remnants of his organization [al Qaeda]. As the arms-control expert Gary Milhollin has put it: "The cash-strapped North Koreans have sold everything [of a military nature] they have produced." Although North Korea might be dissuaded from launching nuclear weapons by the threat of retaliation in kind, such deterrence is no answer to proliferation.

And it may not be a matter of just "two or three" more, in Powell's phrase. We do not know how much uranium the North Koreans have enriched, or what they mean by saying they have another, "more powerful" program. The fuel rods apparently removed from Yongbyon could quickly yield a handful of bombs, and the small reactor being reactivated there

---

1. In spring 2003 the United States led a successful invasion of Iraq to depose Iraqi leader Saddam Hussein, who was thought to be producing weapons of mass destruction.

could produce another one or two a year. Completion of the two much larger reactors whose construction was suspended in 1994 would supply the North Koreans or their customers with enough fissionable material annually for dozens more bombs. If we cannot stop them, as we have been trying without success to do for some twenty years, we face the prospect of North Korea's becoming, in [chairman of the Defense Policy Board] Richard Perle's phrase, the "nuclear breadbasket of the world"—or at least of the underworld of failed states and terror bands.

Here, then, is an especially terrifying version of the nightmare of which President Bush has spoken since [the terrorist attacks of] September 11, 2001: weapons of mass destruction, further along in their development than those of Saddam Hussein, no less likely to be supplied to terrorists, and in the possession of a country, about which our sources of information are even weaker than in the case of Iraq.

How did America get into this fix?

How did we get into this fix? The story is both tedious and instructive—and, for anyone who has followed the cat-and-mouse game played by Saddam Hussein over the last twelve years—eerily evocative.

North Korea began to construct a nuclear reactor large enough to produce material for weapons in 1979. In 1985, in conjunction with a deal for a reactor, and under pressure from us, the Soviets persuaded their then-ally to sign the non-proliferation treaty. But sighs of relief proved premature.

North Korea began to construct a nuclear reactor large enough to produce material for weapons in 1979.

Nations that join the NPT have another eighteen months in which to sign a "safeguards agreement" with the IAEA, under which they openly declare their nuclear programs and arrange for inspectors to monitor them. Eighteen months passed, and then an extension of another eighteen, and still North Korea did not sign. Finally, in 1989, it announced a condition—it would sign if South Korea agreed to turn the entire Korean peninsula into a nuclear-free zone. That same year, while this ostensible olive branch hung in the air, Pyongyang was busily advancing its nuclear program, shutting down its reactor for two to three months in order, apparently, to remove fuel rods for reprocessing into weapons material (while continuing to deny any such nefarious intention).

Over the next two years, Pyongyang stonewalled, insisting not only that the entire peninsula be "denuclearized" but that the annual U.S.–South Korean military exercise called "Team Spirit" be canceled and that the U.S. pledge not to attack the North. Although Washington initially resisted these demands—on the grounds that the tactical nuclear weapons we maintained in the South constituted an essential counterweight to North Korea's overwhelming artillery presence along the demilitarized zone (DMZ) between the two Koreas—gradually it yielded. In

September 1991, President George H.W. Bush announced the withdrawal of all U.S. nuclear weapons from the South.

It did not help; quite the contrary. North Korea first said it would not permit inspections until the withdrawal had actually been completed, and then declared it would permit such inspections only if the U.S. allowed inspections of its own military facilities in the South. By December 1991, the Bush administration had said yes to this, too.

Meanwhile, South Korea, its habitual toughness vitiated by America's string of concessions, had launched its own policy of conciliation. In November, the government in Seoul unilaterally renounced the manufacture, possession, or use of nuclear or chemical weapons, and in December it signed a nonaggression pact that made no mention of the North's nuclear programs but included pledges of economic exchange that would disproportionately benefit the North. The next month, January 1992, the two Koreas agreed to ban nuclear weapons from the peninsula—and still North Korea had not signed a "safeguards" agreement.

Pyongyang repeatedly rebuffed Blix's requests for access [to nuclear facilities].

To sweeten the pot further, President Bush now announced cancellation of the annual Team Spirit exercises. Sure enough, on January 31, Pyongyang signed an inspection plan with the IAEA—but declared immediately thereafter that the plan would have to be ratified by its "legislature," a process slated to take several months. While these deliberations, such as they were, were under way, U.S. surveillance cameras observed convoys of tracks hauling things away from known nuclear sites; in February, following testimony by CIA director Robert Gates to Congress, the *New York Times* reported "a growing consensus in the Bush administration" that North Korea "remains intent on continuing its nuclear-weapons program."

Pyongyang did eventually ratify the accord. But its formal declaration to the IAEA failed to specify how much plutonium it had produced, and its list of nuclear facilities omitted an all-important reprocessing plant at Yongbyon, a multistory facility the length of two football fields that Pyongyang labeled a "radiochemical laboratory." When the director of the IAEA—it was Hans Blix—protested, Pyongyang allowed the plant to be added to the list, at the same time floating the suggestion that it would give up the facility entirely if the West would supply it with light-water reactors, which it said it wanted in order to generate electricity. (The claim that its nuclear program was intended solely to provide electricity was put forward many times by the North, although it never took steps to link any of its reactors to the nation's electricity grid.)

Another dispute developed over two other sites at Yongbyon that U.S. intelligence believed were being used for nuclear waste. One was a large two-story building around which the Koreans had been observed bulldozing mounds of earth to bury the first story prior to the arrival of inspectors. If the two buildings were indeed waste sites, examination of them might have enabled inspectors to deduce how much plutonium North Korea had reprocessed and thus how many bombs it had produced.

But Pyongyang repeatedly rebuffed Blix's requests for access. The quarrel culminated in March 1993 with North Korea's announcement that it was withdrawing from the NPT.

Clinton era failures

By now the Clinton era had begun. Following the example of the Bush administration, the Clinton team likewise tried to lure North Korea with incentives, offering to allow inspection of U.S. military facilities in South Korea and pledging noninterference in the North's internal affairs. In exchange, Pyongyang agreed to "suspend" its withdrawal from the NPT, while adamantly continuing to disallow inspections of the suspected waste sites. By now, indeed, it was also refusing access to the seven declared nuclear sites that inspectors had been permitted to visit the previous year. And, just to reinforce the sense of menace, on the day after suspending its withdrawal from the NPT it test-fired a mid-range ballistic missile capable of reaching Japanese cities with a chemical or nuclear payload.

In November 1993, President [Bill] Clinton underscored the gravity of the threat. "North Korea," he said, "cannot be allowed to develop a nuclear bomb. We have to be very firm about it." Yet in the next weeks administration officials also said they were prepared to offer new inducements, in particular by placing on the back burner the urgent demand for inspection of the two suspected waste sites. As one State Department official told the *Washington Post*, the administration's new strategy was to "walk softly and carry a big carrot."

Not big enough, apparently. The next month, December 1993, the *New York Times* reported a CIA assessment concluding that North Korea already possessed one or two nuclear bombs. But far from stiffening Washington's attitude, this seemed to breed a mood of submission. Soon, a White House spokesman was saying the President had "misspoken" about not allowing North Korea to have nuclear weapons, and Washington even tried to soften the approach of the IAEA, then as now a UN agency hardly known for firmness, by discouraging it from bringing Pyongyang's nonfeasance to the Security Council.

A White House spokesman was saying the President had "misspoken" about not allowing North Korea to have nuclear weapons.

After another round of diplomacy, and in exchange for fresh American concessions, the two sides announced a new deal allowing inspections of declared sites to go forward. (The two undeclared waste sites were now so far on the back burner as to be entirely lost from view.) The returning inspectors found the seals they had left on equipment broken; when they tried to take samples from the reprocessing plant to see what had been done, the North Koreans sent them packing. "This time," a Clinton official told the *Times*, "the North went too far. There are no more carrots." "We are going to stop them," said Defense Secretary William Perry resolutely. "I'd rather face [the risk of war] than face the risk of even greater catastrophe two or three years from now." But within a couple of weeks, Secretary of State Warren Christopher was explaining that the U.S. was willing to negotiate for another six months, and Perry pulled in his horns.

The fix we are in is the fruit of a long pattern of appeasement and of North Korea's canny manipulation of our illusions and fears.

In May 1994, North Korea brought matters to a head by announcing that it was removing spent fuel from its Yongbyon reactor without international monitoring. Removal of the 8,000 fuel rods posed a double whammy. If inspectors could not sample them, there would be no way of tracing how much plutonium had previously been recovered from the reactor. Plus, additional plutonium could now be taken, presumably enough to make several more bombs. At this point, the IAEA declared that it could no longer assure that North Korea's program was not being used for weapons, and North Korea, trumpeting defiance, resigned its membership in the agency. Washington began eliciting support for economic sanctions and beefed up its military forces in the region. Talk of war was in the air.

Jimmy Carter's failed efforts

But the threat of conflagration was laid to rest by an astonishing diplomatic intervention by former President Jimmy Carter. An outspoken critic of U.S. policy for being too hard on North Korea, Carter flew to Pyongyang for some personal diplomacy with Kim Il Sung, a ruthless dictator who had been handpicked for his job by [Soviet leader Joseph] Stalin himself. Where previous Western visitors to Pyongyang had described a city darkened by power shortages, with little commerce and a populace terrified to be seen conversing with foreigners, Carter reported a bustling metropolis with shops much like the "Wal-Mart in Americus, Georgia," neon lights that reminded him of "Times Square," and a population that was "friendly and open."

The wonders of the city were but a prelude to what Carter found when he came face to face with Kim. The dictator, he discovered, was "revered" and "treated as a combination of George Washington, Thomas Jefferson, and Abe Lincoln." Carter also found Kim "very friendly toward Christianity." Although now in his eighties, Kim was "vigorous, intelligent, surprisingly well-informed," and "very frank." What is more, by showing Kim proper respect, Carter had achieved a "miracle": the basis for a new agreement.

In the ensuing months, Washington and Pyongyang reached an "agreed framework" under which North Korea would freeze its existing plutonium program. In exchange, it was to receive two light-water reactors and—pending their completion—500,000 metric tons of heavy oil annually, amounting to about 40 percent of the country's fuel consumption. The reactors and the oil were to come as gifts, paid for by South Korea, Japan, the U.S., and Europe. In addition, various trade and diplomatic restrictions, the legacy of North Korea's invasion of the South decades earlier and of terrorist attacks that had continued into the 1980's, were to be lifted.

In the U.S., the deal came in for a fair amount of criticism. It seemed to reward Pyongyang for its defiance of the NPT, thereby setting a dangerous precedent. It left the plutonium facilities intact and spent fuel inside the country, thus allowing the program to be restarted easily. Moreover, the light-water reactors could themselves produce plutonium, and although in some respects less conducive to a weapons program, they were far from weapons-proof. Indeed, Washington was at that very moment trying to dissuade Russia from supplying such reactors to Iran.

> *"Diplomacy" might indeed get us a deal; but what would it be worth?*

But the deal was also defended. For the time being, it had stopped North Korea's program in its tracks. And in the long run, it was said, there was reason to hope that the bankrupt North Korean regime would collapse before the light-water reactors were up and running and producing plutonium, a process that was estimated at about ten years. "Five years from now, North Korea is not going to be there," the *Washington Post* quoted a senior Defense Department official as saying; the paper added that by then, according to intelligence assessments, "North Korea's economic troubles could topple its leadership and force unification with South Korea."

Today, more than eight years later, North Korea is still there, and is still ruled by the Kim dynasty, Kim Il Sung having been succeeded upon his death by his son, Kim Jong Il. The merits of the "agreed framework" are a moot point. Pyongyang was cheating on it all along, the inexorably mounting evidence to this effect having culminated in North Korea's momentous proclamation of last October.

Diplomacy will fail

Given this history, only a fraction of whose tortuous windings and humiliating frustrations I have been able to convey, it is nothing short of astonishing that today, political leaders like Jimmy Carter and even Senator Joseph Lieberman, as well as columnists like the *New York Times*'s Paul Krugman, the *Washington Post*'s Richard Cohen, and *Newsweek*'s Fareed Zakaria, rushed to lay the entire crisis at the door of George W. Bush. But so they did. In describing North Korea as part of the "axis of evil" in his 2002 State of the Union Address,[2] and otherwise rebuffing it, the new President, or so the line went, had driven Pyongyang to misbehave. "Put yourself in Kim Jong Il's shoes," pleaded Krugman. According to this logic, the new crisis consisted not of North Korea's nuclear-weapons program, which had commenced years before Bush came to office, but of the fact that we had somehow coerced the North Koreans into confessing to it.

2. In his speech Bush called Iraq, Iran, and North Korea an "axis of evil," threatening global security.

Yet far from being the fault of this administration, the fix we are in is the fruit of a long pattern of appeasement and of North Korea's canny manipulation of our illusions and fears. Once we discovered that Pyongyang was indeed building a nuclear reactor, we spent five or six years getting it to sign the NPT, then another seven years securing its signature to a "safeguards" agreement, then three more vainly trying to induce it to abide by that agreement. We finally abandoned the effort in favor of a "framework," which eight years later it admitted it had been disregarding all along. At the core of this pathetic tale was our reluctance to consider that the goal of the North Koreans' nuclear-weapons program was to possess nuclear weapons—and that diplomatic and economic incentives to avert this goal might be of no avail. In place of a frank recognition of this reality, we substituted our vain hopes that North Korea's rulers could be softened by concessions, and that what they really wanted was economic aid, political legitimacy, and "respect."

How, then, do we get out of the fix? Even after the disclosure in late January of the apparent removal of 8,000 fuel rods from Yongbyon, the Bush team has continued to insist that the matter will be solved by diplomacy, and has appealed to Russia and China for help. Jimmy Carter has urged us to offer new incentives to Pyongyang, as has former Secretary of Defense William S. Cohen and commentators like the *Times*'s Nicholas Kristof and Bill Keller. "More for more," Keller has proposed, meaning sweeping nuclear disarmament by North Korea in exchange for a much richer package of economic and political benefits than it has been offered before.

Ultimately, the world is likely to be safe with North Korea . . . only through the demise of its current government.

But the problem with all of these proposals, quite apart from the fact that they seem to ignore our experience, is that even if we struck a grand bargain there would be no way of knowing that the other side was keeping its word. "Diplomacy" might indeed get us a deal; but what would it be worth?

The North Koreans are master diggers. The DMZ is said to be honeycombed with tunnels through which vast quantities of military personnel and equipment can invade the South in any new Korean war. (Some of these tunnels have been discovered and closed; no one doubts that many undiscovered ones remain.) As best we can make out, the North Koreans have also built underground nuclear reactors, plutonium-reprocessing plants, and uranium-enrichment facilities—and who knows what else? Iraq, as we discovered after the 1991 war, had built an entire nuclear program right under the nose of the IAEA, all the while complying with every inspection request. The hilly terrain of North Korea is more conducive to concealment than the flat sands of Iraq, and North Korea's is a much more closed society. As helpless as inspectors have been in finding Iraq's weapons, they would be more helpless still in North Korea.

Other fail-prone proposals

In contrast to those who want to offer new inducements, several tougher-minded commentators have called for "isolating" North Korea through UN sanctions. But it is doubtful that even the strictest sanctions would make a dent, since North Korea is already, by its own choosing, one of the world's most isolated nations. It is even more doubtful that the UN Security Council would apply the strictest sanctions.

Only China has the leverage to squeeze North Korea hard, since, now that we have suspended our oil shipments, North Korea depends almost entirely on that country for fuel. But China has so far insisted, as it has always done, that our issues with Pyongyang be resolved through "dialogue."

The preservation of all we hold dear will require unillusioned clarity, vigilance, courage—and, it is to be feared, sacrifice.

Another proposal, this one by [columnist] Charles Krauthammer, is to help Japan to become a nuclear power, on the reasoning that the threat of a nuclear Japan is the only way to pressure China to turn the screws on North Korea. Clever though it is, this leads to the same problem as the proposals for wooing Kim with new inducements. Any diplomatic solution whether it is secured by twisting Kim's arm or by caressing his cheek—ends up in a deal that has to be verified, and there can be no confidence in our ability to verify the North's nuclear disarmament. We do not know what weapons or nuclear programs it has, and there is no sure way to find out so long as Kim rules the country.

The same fatal flaw sinks another proposal, by [editor of the *National Review*] John O'Sullivan, for an "inglorious deal" whereby North Korea would receive various benefits and be allowed to keep its nuclear capabilities in exchange for ceasing to sell to others. The logic of focusing on the proliferation threat is admittedly compelling. In itself, a nuclear-armed North Korea might be less dangerous than a nuclear-armed Iraq. It would be easier for us to protect North Korea's few neighbors, and unlike in the case of Iraq, whose military might ramifies throughout the Middle Eastern and Arab worlds, North Korea influences almost nobody. But would a commitment not to transfer nuclear components be any more verifiable than a commitment not to develop them? Smuggling is an easier art than tunneling, and if North Koreans can hide entire reactors, they can surely hide the passage of a few bombs.

The Heritage Foundation's John Tkacik has suggested tackling the proliferation problem by means of an air and sea embargo of North Korea. Perhaps this would work, but one fiendish thing about nuclear material is that it is not large. As a rule of thumb, the IAEA says, eight kilograms of plutonium are required to make a bomb. Add to that the shielding needed to transport the stuff, and you still can move it in a small airplane or boat. It is doubtful we have the technical means to spot and interdict all such craft. Moreover, any such effort would require Chinese cooperation.

War may be necessary

Ultimately, the world is likely to be safe with North Korea, as with Iraq, only through the demise of its current government. In 1994, we believed that the Kim dynasty was likely to fall of its own dead weight, just as we thought that Saddam Hussein would fall in 1991 after his humiliating defeat in the "mother of all battles." Predicting the fall of dictators is clearly a chancy business. In the hope of opening fissures in the closed polity of North Korea, a group of neoconservative intellectuals, including Max Kampelman, R. James Woolsey, and Penn Kemble, have suggested adding human-rights issues to the diplomatic agenda. A fine idea; but the only way to assure regime change in North Korea is through military action.

But war, we have been told by numerous analysts as well as implicitly by the Bush administration, is "unthinkable." The North Koreans have hundreds of thousands of soldiers and thousands of artillery pieces arrayed in and around the DMZ. Their shells can reach Seoul. Any war would mean the deaths of many thousands of South Korean soldiers and civilians, and many of the 37,000 American troops stationed on the front lines. This is not even to mention whatever harm the North might manage to inflict with its nuclear devices.

Horrible, war would be. But to say that it is unthinkable is once again to hide our head in the sand. Pyongyang itself suffers under no such illusions and no such inhibitions. For its part, it insists that economic sanctions will be taken as an act of war, implying that it would respond with military strikes. Indeed, far from having viewed war with us as unthinkable, the North has calculated its demands on us over the years—that we remove our tactical nuclear weapons, that we persuade the South Koreans to forswear nuclear weapons of their own, that we cancel joint military exercises with Seoul—precisely in order to weaken our ability to resist its own military power. These demands we have systematically granted.

Not only does the North's belligerence leave us no choice but to "think" about war, we cannot exclude the possibility of initiating military action ourselves. Part of the cause of our present predicament is that we ruled out the use of force at earlier points in this saga—when, however painful, it would have been less costly than today. And today it may be less costly than a few years from now, when North Korea will have dozens of nuclear weapons and long-range missiles (it has tested one that could reach Alaska) or when it will have shared them with al Qaeda and others.

The frailty of "parchment barriers"

Is there anything to be learned from the appalling choices we find ourselves facing? The *New York Times* editorialized in January that Pyongyang's confession had "blown apart the Bush administration's months-long effort to portray Saddam Hussein as uniquely dangerous." The implication was that the North Korean menace spoke against the policy of disarming Iraq by force. What it really did was the opposite. It illustrated how such threats grow ever worse if they are not dealt with resolutely. Contrary to those who airily put their trust in "containment," it gave us a glimpse into how much more dangerous the world would be if we allowed Iraq to join North Korea in the nuclear club. Since appeasement has only emboldened the North Koreans, perhaps making an example of Saddam Hussein may take some of the wind out of their nuclear sails.

In short, our experience with North Korea confirms anew the folly of appeasement and the frailty of "parchment barriers"—not to mention the wisdom of missile defense. Above all, it points up the error of lowering our guard. Since the cold war ended, we were living in something of a fool's paradise. All of the conflicts in which we were embroiled after the fall of Communism—Kuwait, Bosnia, Somalia, Haiti, Kosovo—were minor in comparison to our decades-long tussle with the Soviet empire. Although the issues were real, the dangers were always contingent, and we enjoyed a wide margin for error. Accordingly, we progressively reduced the size of our military and our spending on weapons until we abandoned, first in practice and then in doctrine, the capacity, to wage wars simultaneously on two fronts. The result was, and is, that our ability to confront North Korea is constrained by our mobilization around Iraq—a fact that by itself helps to explain the brazenness of the North Koreans.

With the fall of the Soviet empire, as Francis Fukuyama eloquently explained more than a dozen years ago, no ideology remained to rival our own. Neither was there any foe on the horizon that could hope to vanquish us. Modern weapons, however, endow even a minor power with the capability of wreaking terrible damage, and of killing Americans in larger numbers than Hitler. . . . That such weapons can be fielded by North Korea, a country so miserable that infinitely more of is people are eating grass than are shopping at "Wal-Marts," underscores how far removed we are from the old calculus in which military potency derived from industrial might.

The ideological competitors with democracy and capitalism have indeed faded. But these were mostly phenomena of the 20th century. What has remained is something older and deeper: the atavistic impulses of self-aggrandizement and nihilism. How else to classify the motor force behind the dynasty-Communism of the Kims, the Baathism-cum-Islamism of Saddam, the twisted preachings of bin Laden? When there are no longer powerful men like these, then we may truly begin to speak of the end of history. Until then, the preservation of all we hold dear will require unillusioned clarity, vigilance, courage—and, it is to be feared, sacrifice.

8

The 2003 War in Iraq Increased Nuclear Security

Dick Cheney

Dick Cheney, U.S. vice president under George W. Bush, was in office when America went to war in Iraq in 2003.

Critics complain that the United States started the 2003 war against Iraq without direct provocation, an act they consider a breach of international law. However, waiting until Iraqi leader Saddam Hussein and the terrorists he supported attacked the United States with weapons of mass destruction would have had disastrous consequences. Weapons inspections conducted after the war have revealed extensive efforts by Hussein to build chemical, biological, and nuclear weapons, which could have been used against the United States or sold to anti-American terrorists. The war in Iraq has rid the Middle East of a brutal tyrant and fostered global peace and security.

Editor's Note: In spring 2003 the United States led an invasion of Iraq and deposed Iraqi leader Saddam Hussein. The war was part of a larger war on terrorism, begun after Middle East terrorists killed approximately three thousand people in New York City, Washington, D.C., and Pennsylvania on September 11, 2001.

For most of this year [2003], the attention of the world has centered on Iraq, from the final ultimatum to [Iraqi leader] Saddam Hussein last March, to the removal of his regime and on up to the present, as we continue to battle with Saddam loyalists and foreign terrorists.

The center of the war on terror

Iraq has become the central front in the war on terror. It was crucial that we enforce the U.N. Security Council resolutions [which required Iraq to destroy its weapons of mass destruction]. Now, having liberated that country, it is crucial that we keep our word to the Iraqi people, helping them to

Dick Cheney, address before the Heritage Foundation, Washington, DC, October 10, 2003.

build a secure country and a democratic government. And we will do so.

Our mission in Iraq is a great undertaking and part of a larger mission that the United States accepted now more than two years ago. [The terrorist attacks of] September 11th, 2001 changed everything for this country. We came to recognize our vulnerability to the threats of the new era. We saw the harm that 19 evil men could do, armed with little more than airline tickets and box cutters and driven by a philosophy of hatred.

We lost some 3,000 innocent lives that morning in scarcely two hours time.

Since 9/11, we've learned much more about what these enemies intend for us. One member of Al Qaida said 9/11 was the beginning of the end of America. And we know to a certainty that terrorists are doing everything they can to gain even deadlier means of striking us. From the training manuals we found in the caves of Afghanistan to the interrogations of terrorists that we capture, we have learned of their ambitions to develop or acquire chemical, biological or nuclear weapons.

And if terrorists ever do acquire that capability, on their own or with help from a terror regime, they will use it without the slightest constraint of reason or morality.

That possibility, the ultimate nightmare, could bring devastation to our country on a scale we have never experienced. Instead of losing thousands of lives, we might lose tens of thousands or even hundreds of thousands of lives in a single day of horror.

Remember what we saw on the morning of 9/11. And knowing the nature of these enemies, we have as clear a responsibility as to ever fall to government. We must do everything in our power to keep terrorists from ever acquiring weapons of mass destruction.

A shift in national security policy

This great and urgent responsibility has required [a] shift [in] national security policy. The strategy of deterrence which served us so well during the decades of the Cold War will no longer do. Our terrorist enemy has no country to defend, no assets to destroy in order to discourage an attack.

Strategies of containment will not assure our security either. There's no containing a terrorist who will commit suicide for the purposes of mass slaughter. There's also no containing a terrorist state that secretly passes along deadly weapons to a terrorist network.

There is only one way to protect ourselves against catastrophic terrorist violence, and that is to destroy the terrorists before they can launch further attacks against the United States.

Terrorists are doing everything they can to gain even deadlier means of striking us.

For many years prior to 9/11, it was the terrorists who were on the offensive. We treated their repeated attacks against Americans as isolated incidents and answered, if at all, on an ad hoc basis and rarely in a systematic way.

There was the attack on the Marine barracks in Beirut, 1983, killing 241 men; the bombing of the World Trade Center in 1993; five more murders when the Saudi National Guard Training Center in Riyadh was struck in 1995; the killings at Khobar Towers in 1996; the East Africa embassy bombings in 1998; and in 2000, the attack on the USS *Cole*.

There was a tendency to treat incidents like these as individual criminal acts to be handled primarily through law enforcement. Ramzi Yousef, who perpetrated the first attack on the World Trade Center, is the best case in point.

A good defense is not enough. We're going after the terrorists wherever they plot and plan.

The U.S. government tracked him down, arrested him and got a conviction. After he was sent off to serve a 240-year sentence, some might have thought, "Case closed." But the case was not closed. The leads were not successfully followed. The dots were not adequately connected. The threat was not recognized for what it was.

For Al Qaida [the group responsible for September 11], the World Trade Center attack in 1993 was part of a sustained campaign. Behind that one man, Ramzi Yousef, was a growing network with operatives inside and outside the United States, waging war against our country. For us, that war started on 9/11. For them, it started years ago, when [Al Qaida leader] Osama bin Laden declared war on the United States.

In 1996, Khalid Sheik Mohammed, the mastermind of 9/11 and the uncle of Ramzi Yousef, first proposed to bin Laden that they use hijacked airliners to attack targets in the U.S. During this period, thousands of terrorists were trained at Al Qaida camps in Afghanistan.

Since September 11th, the terrorists have continued their attacks in Riyadh, Casablanca, Mombasa, Bali, Jakarta, Najaf and Baghdad. Against this kind of determined, organized, ruthless enemy, America requires a new strategy, not merely to prosecute a series of crimes, but to conduct a global campaign against the terror network.

The strategy's key elements

Our strategy has several key elements. We've strengthened our defenses here at home, organizing the government to protect the homeland. But a good defense is not enough. We're going after the terrorists wherever they plot and plan.

Of those known to be directly involved in organizing the attacks of 9/11, most are now in custody or confirmed dead. The leadership of Al Qaida has sustained heavy losses; they will sustain more.

We're also dismantling the financial networks that support terror, a vital step never before taken. The hidden bank accounts, the front groups, the phony charities are being discovered and the assets seized to starve terrorists of the money that makes it possible for them to operate.

Our government is also working closely with intelligence services all over the globe, including those of governments not traditionally considered friends of the United States. And we are applying the Bush doctrine: Any person or government that supports, protects or harbors terrorists is complicit in the murder of the innocent and will be held to account.

The first to see this doctrine in application were the Taliban, who ruled Afghanistan by violence while turning the country into a training camp for terrorists. With fine allies at our side, we took down the regime and shut down the Al Qaida camps.

Our work there continues, confronting Taliban and Al Qaida remnants, training a new Afghan army and providing security as the new government takes shape. Under President Karzai's leadership, and with the help of our coalition, the Afghan people are building a decent and just society, a nation fully joined in the war on terror.

Reasons for war on Iraq

In Iraq [in 2003], we took another essential step in the war on terror. The United States and our allies rid the Iraqi people of a murderous dictator and rid the world of a menace to our future peace and security.

Saddam had a lengthy history of reckless and sudden aggression. He cultivated ties to terror, hosting the Abu Nidal organization, supporting terrorists, making payments to the families of suicide bombers in Israel. He also had an established relationship with Al Qaida, providing training to Al Qaida members in the areas of poisons, gases, making conventional bombs.

Saddam built, possessed and used weapons of mass destruction [WMD].

He refused or evaded all international demands to account for those weapons.

The United States and our allies . . . rid the world of a menace to our future peace and security.

Twelve years of diplomacy, more than a dozen Security Council resolutions, hundreds of U.N. weapons inspectors, thousands of flights to enforce the no-fly zones and even strikes against military targets in Iraq, all of these measures were tried to compel Saddam Hussein's compliance with the terms of the 1991 Gulf War cease-fire. All of these measures failed.

Last October [2002], the United States Congress voted overwhelming to authorize the use of force in Iraq.

Last November, the U.N. Security Council passed a unanimous resolution finding Iraq in material breach of its obligations and vowing serious consequences in the event Saddam Hussein did not fully and immediately comply. When Saddam Hussein failed even then to comply, our coalition acted to deliver those serious consequences.

In that effort, the American military acted with speed and precision and skill. Once again, our men and women in uniform have served with honor, reflecting great credit on themselves and on the United States of America.

In the post-9/11 era, certain risks are unacceptable. The United States made our position clear: We could not accept the grave danger of Saddam

Hussein and his terrorist allies turning weapons of mass destruction against us or our friends and allies.

The Kay report

And gradually, we are learning the details of his hidden weapons program. This work is being carried out under the direction of Dr. David Kay, a respected scientist and former U.N. inspector, who is leading the weapons search in Iraq.

Dr. Kay's team faces an enormous task: They have yet to examine more than 100 large conventional weapons arsenals, some of which cover areas larger than 50 square miles.

Finding comparatively small volumes of extremely deadly materials hidden in these vast stockpiles will be time-consuming and difficult. Yet Dr. Kay and his team are making progress and have compiled an interim report, portions of which were declassified [in October 2003].

Let me read to you a couple of passages from Dr. Kay's testimony to Congress, which deserve closer attention.

He notes, quote, "Iraq's WMD programs spanned more than two decades, involved thousands of people, billions of dollars, and were elaborately shielded by security and deception operations that continued even beyond the end of Operation Iraqi Freedom," end quote.

Dr. Kay further stated, "We have discovered dozens of WMD-related program activities and significant amounts of equipment that Iraq concealed from the United Nations during the inspections that began in late 2002.

"The discovery of these deliberate concealment efforts have come about, both through the admissions of Iraqi scientists and officials, concerning information they deliberately withheld, as well as through physical evidence of equipment and activities that the Iraq Survey Group has discovered should have been declared to the United Nations."

The evidence

Among the items Dr. Kay and his team have already identified are the following:

- A clandestine network of laboratories and safe houses within the Iraqi intelligence service. They contained equipment suitable for continuing chemical and biological weapons research.
- A prison laboratory complex, possibly used in human testing of biological weapons agents that Iraqi officials were explicitly ordered not to declare to the United Nations.
- Reference strains of biological organisms concealed in a scientist's home, one of which can be used to produce biological weapons [BW].
- New research on BW-applicable agents brucella and Congo-Crimean hemorrhagic fever. And continuing work on ricin and aflatoxin which had not been declared to the United Nations.
- Documents and equipment hidden in scientists' homes that would have been useful in resuming uranium enrichment by centrifuge and electromagnetic isotope separation.
- A line of unmanned aerial vehicles, not fully declared, and an ad-

mission that they had been tested out to a range of 500 kilometers: 350 kilometers beyond the legal limit imposed by the U.N. after the Gulf War.

- Plans and advanced design work for new long-range ballistic and cruise missiles with ranges capable of striking targets throughout the Middle East, which were prohibited by the U.N. and which Saddam sought to conceal from U.N. weapons inspectors.
- Clandestine attempts between late 1999 and 2002 to obtain from North Korea technology related to 1,300-kilometer-range ballistic missiles, 300-kilometer-range anti-ship cruise missiles and other prohibited military equipment.

Now, ladies and gentlemen, each and every one of these findings confirms a material breach by the former Iraqi regime of U.N. Security Council Resolution 1441. Taken together, they constitute a massive breach of that unanimously passed resolution and provide a compelling case for the use of force against Saddam Hussein.

Critics' claims

Even as more evidence is found of Saddam's weapons programs, critics of our action in Iraq continue to voice other objections. And the arguments they make are helping to frame the most important debate of the post-9/11 era. Some claim we should not have acted because the threat from Saddam Hussein was not imminent. Yet, as the president has said, "Since when have terrorists and tyrants announced their intention, politely putting us on notice before they strike?"

I would remind the critics of the fundamental case the president has made since September 11th. Terrorist enemies of our country hope to strike us with the most lethal weapons known to man and it would be reckless in the extreme to rule out action and save our worries until the day they strike.

As the president told Congress earlier [in 2003], if threats from terrorists and terror states are permitted to fully emerge, all actions, all words and all recriminations would come too late. That is the debate. That is the choice set before the American people.

And as long as George W. Bush is president of the United States, this country will not permit gathering threats to become certain tragedies.

We could not accept the grave danger of Saddam Hussein . . . turning weapons of mass destruction against us.

Critics of our national security policy have also argued that to confront a gathering threat is simply to stir up hostility. In the case of Saddam Hussein, his hostility to our country long predates 9/11 and America's war on terror.

In the case of the Al Qaida terrorists, their hostility has long been evident. And year after year, the terrorists only grew bolder in the absence of forceful response from America and other nations. Weakness and drift and vacillation in the face of danger invite attacks. Strength and resolve and decisive action defeat attacks before they can arrive on our soil.

Another criticism we hear is that the United States, when its security is threatened, may not act without unanimous international consent. Under this view, even in the face of a specific stated agreed-upon danger, the mere objection of even one foreign government would be sufficient to prevent us from acting.

It would be reckless in the extreme to rule out action and save our worries until the day [terrorists] strike.

This view reflects a deep confusion about the requirements of our national security. Though often couched in high-sounding terms of unity and cooperation, it is a prescription for perpetual disunity and obstructionism.

In practice, it would prevent our own country from acting with friends and allies, even in the most urgent circumstance. To accept the view that action by America and our allies can be stopped by the objection of foreign governments that may not feel threatened is to confer undue power on them while leaving the rest of us powerless to act in our own defense.

Yet we continue to hear this attitude and arguments in our own country. So often, and so conveniently, it amounts to a policy of doing exactly nothing.

Working with friends and allies

In Afghanistan, in Iraq, on every front in the war on terror, the United States has cooperated with friends and allies and with others who recognize the common threat we face. More than 50 countries are contributing to peace and stability in Iraq today, including most of the world's democracies, and more than 70 are with us in Afghanistan.

The United States is committed to multilateral action wherever possible, yet this commitment does not require us to stop everything and neglect our own defense merely on the say so of a single foreign government.

This is the debate before the American people and it is of more than academic interest. It comes down to a choice between action that assures our security and inaction that allows dangers to grow. And we can see the consequences of these choices in real events. The contrast is greatest on the ground in Iraq.

Had the United States been constrained by the objections of some, the regime of Saddam Hussein would still rule Iraq, his statues would still stand, his sons would still be running the secret police, dissidents would still be in prison, the apparatus of torture and rape would still be in place, and the mass graves would be undiscovered.

We must never forget the kind of man who ran that country and the depravity of his regime.

[In September 2003] Bernard Kerik, former police commissioner of

New York returned from Iraq after spending four months helping to activate and stand up a new national police force. Bernie Kerik tells of many things he saw, including the videos of interrogations in which the victim is blown apart by a hand grenade. Another video, as he describes it, shows and I quote, "Saddam sitting in an office allowing two Doberman Pinchers to eat alive a general because he did not trust his loyalty," end quote.

Those who declined to support the liberation of Iraq would not deny the evil of Saddam Hussein's regime. They must concede, however, that had their own advice been followed, that regime would rule Iraq today.

President Bush declined the course of inaction and the results are there for all to see. The torture chambers are empty, the prisons for children are closed, the murders of innocents have been exposed and their mass graves have been uncovered. The regime is gone, never to return. And despite difficulties we knew would occur, the Iraqi people prefer liberty and hope to tyranny and fear.

Had we followed the counsel of inaction, the Iraqi regime would still be a . . . destabilizing force in the Middle East.

Our coalition is helping them to build a secure, hopeful and self-governing nation which will stand as an example of freedom to all the Middle East. We are rebuilding more than 1,000 schools, supplying and reopening hospitals, rehabilitating power plants, water and sanitation facilities, bridges and airports.

Positive trends

We are training Iraqi police, border guards and a new army, so that the Iraqi people can assume full responsibility for their own security.

Iraq now has its own governing council, has appointed interim government ministers and is moving toward the drafting of a new constitution and free elections.

The contrast of visions is evident, as well, throughout the region. Had we followed the counsel of inaction, the Iraqi regime would still be a menace to its neighbors and a destabilizing force in the Middle East. Today, because we acted, Iraq stands to be a force for good in the Middle East.

Comparing both sides of the debate, we can see certain consequences for the world, beyond the Middle East, consequences with direct implications for our own security.

If Saddam Hussein were in power today, there would still be active terror camps in Iraq, the regime would still be allowing terrorist leaders into the country and this ally of terrorists would still have a hidden biological weapons program capable of producing deadly agents on short notice.

There would be today, as there was six months ago, the prospect of the Iraqi dictator providing weapons of mass destruction, or the means to make them, to terrorists for the purpose of attacking America.

Today, we do not face this prospect. There are terrorists in Iraq, yet there is no dictator to protect them and we are dealing with them, one by one. Terrorists have gathered in that country and there they will be defeated. We are fighting this evil in Iraq so we do not have to fight it on the streets of our own cities.

The current debate over America's national security policy is the most consequential since the early days of the Cold War and the emergence of a bipartisan commitment to face the evils of communism.

All of us now look back with respect and gratitude on the great decisions that set America on the path to victory in the Cold War and kept us on that path through nine presidencies.

I believe that, one day, scholars and historians will look back on our time and pay tribute to our 43rd president who has both called upon and exemplified the courage and perseverance of the American people.

In this period of extraordinary danger, President Bush has made clear America's purposes in the world and our determination to overcome the threats to our liberty and our lives.

Sometimes history presents clear and stark choices—we have come to such a moment. Those who bear the responsibility for making those choices for America must understand that while action will always carry cost, measured in effort and sacrifice, inaction carries heavy costs of its own.

As in the years of the Cold War, much is asked of us and much rides on our actions. A watching world is depending on the United States of America.

Only America has the might and the will to lead the world through a time of peril toward greater security and peace.

And as we've done before, we accept the great mission that history has given us.

9

The 2003 War in Iraq Did Not Increase Nuclear Security

Joseph Cirincione

Joseph Cirincione is project director at the Carnegie Endowment for International Peace, an organization that conducts research on international affairs and U.S. foreign policy.

Despite assertions from the Bush administration that the 2003 war in Iraq was necessary to protect Americans, weapons inspections conducted by the United States after the war have proven that the war was not necessary to maintain global security. Inspectors have uncovered only partially completed weapons programs, evidence that ongoing UN weapons inspections had succeeded in deterring Iraqi leader Saddam Hussein from actively producing biological, chemical, and nuclear weapons. Thousands of lives were sacrificed unnecessarily in this unjust war.

Editor's Note: As a condition of the cessation of hostilities in the 1991 Gulf War, Iraqi leader Saddam Hussein was required by UN resolutions to allow weapons inspectors into his country. In the spring of 2003, after Hussein had failed to cooperate with the inspectors, the United States led a coalition to invade Iraq to depose Hussein. Bush administration officials claimed that the war was necessary to eliminate the possibility that Iraq would target America with weapons of mass destruction or sell them to anti-American terrorists.

The *Boston Globe* discloses that later this month [September 2003] David Kay, head of the 1200-person Iraq Survey Team [charged with uncovering weapons of mass destruction after the 2003 war], will report that although US troops and experts have been unable to find any hard evidence of chemical, biological or nuclear weapons or long-range missiles, they have uncovered a vast conspiracy to deceive United Nations inspectors. According to *Globe* reporter Bryan Bender, Kay "will build a strong, but largely

Joseph Cirincione, "The Kay Report Comedown," *Carnegie Analysis*, September 2, 2003. Copyright © 2003 by the Carnegie Endowment for International Peace, Washington, DC, www.ceip.org. Reproduced by permission.

circumstantial case that [Saddam] Hussein dispersed his weapons programs." Kay will say that he has found evidence of intentions to possibly build such weapons after inspectors left the country.

If all Saddam had were intentions and fragments of [weapons of mass destruction] programs, there was no need for war in March 2003.

If the newspaper is correct, the Kay report will mark the official retreat of US and British pre-war claims. However unintentionally, it will be a direct refutation of official assertions that we had to go to war to prevent Saddam Hussein from using massive stockpiles of chemical and biological weapons and possibly nuclear weapons. Though weapons stocks may still be found, Kay will focus on "dual-use" capabilities that could quickly be reconfigured to manufacture weapons. Though such plans would have been a violation of UN resolutions, this will also be an indication that UN inspections were working. As long as inspectors were in the country, Iraq apparently did not expect to get away with active weapons production.

Pre-war claims

Before the war, officials spoke repeatedly of imminent dangers. President [George W.] Bush said that Iraq had stockpiled biological and chemical weapons, warning explicitly in October 2002 in Cincinnati that Saddam Hussein had "more than 30,000 liters of anthrax and other deadly biological agents" and likely "two to four times that amount." "This is a massive stockpile of biological weapons," he said, "that has never been accounted for and is capable of killing millions." On December 31, he told reporters ominously, "We don't know whether or not he has a [nuclear] bomb."

CIA Director George Tenet told Congress in February, "we will find caches of weapons of mass destruction, absolutely." He also said then that Saddam's "biological-weapons capability is far bigger that it was at the time of the Gulf War, and he has a chemical-weapons capability that he hasn't declared." Secretary of State Colin Powell told the United Nations on February 5 that "Saddam Hussein retains a covert force of up to a few dozen Scud-variant ballistic missiles," and that "U.S. intelligence had tracked the movement of missile warheads filled with biological agent from outside Baghdad to western Iraq." He repeated in March, "We know that in late January, the Iraqi intelligence service transported chemical and biological agents to areas far away from Baghdad, near the Syrian and Turkish borders, in order to conceal them . . . from the prying eyes of inspectors."

On the eve of the war, President Bush told the nation, "Intelligence fathered by this and other governments leaves no doubt that the Iraq regime continues to possess and conceal some of the most lethal weapons ever devised."

In the early days of the war, officials believed the discovery of weapons caches was imminent. "There is no doubt that the regime of Saddam Hussein possesses weapons of mass destruction. As this operation continues, those weapons will be identified, found, along with the people who have produced them and who guard them," said General Tommy Franks on March 23. "I have no doubt we're going to find big stores of weapons of mass destruction," said Defense Policy Board Member Ken Adleman on the same day. Two weeks later, Adleman was still confident, saying on April 10, "People will step forward pretty fast [and identify Iraq's weapons stores]. It should be pretty soon, in the next five days."

The climb down

By May, officials were lowering expectations, talking of "weapons programs" and "capabilities" not weapons themselves. "In some cases, they'll be larger and smaller parts of, say, the missile and delivery systems. I think we're going to find that they had a weapons of mass destruction program. Now, how it was configured and how they intended to use it is part of the hard work that they're going through right now," said Undersecretary of Defense Stephen Cambone on May 7. Undersecretary of Defense Douglas Feith explained to Congress on June 4, "The Iraqis possessed the capability to use chemical weapons, biological weapons" and "they had a program that was aiming toward the development of nuclear weapons."

The Kay report will apparently try to document this program. There will inevitably be criticism of the report for its lack of independence. There is little doubt that the US would be better served if the assessment had been performed by an objective, international agency and not headed by an advocate of the war and an opponent of continuing the UN inspections. Others will point out that the United Nations never intended to leave Iraq free to pursue new weapons programs. The plan was always to establish an on-site verification and monitoring regime after the initial inspections were completed, as indicated by the inspection team's formal name, the United Nations Monitoring, Verification and Inspection Commission (UNMOVIC). The larger point, however, may be that Kay will belabor the obvious.

Prior to 2002, many national and international officials and experts believed that Iraq likely had research programs or some stores of hidden chemical or biological weapons and maintained interest in a program to develop nuclear weapons. The debate that began in 2002 was not over weapons, but over war. The issue was whether Iraq's failure to cooperate fully with United Nations inspections and adequately account for its activities posed such a severe threat as to require military invasion and occupation. There the Kay Report may do more harm to the administration's case. Even if it puts the worst spin on all the available evidence, it may still end up showing that Iraq had far less than anyone imagined, and certainly less than officials claimed.

If all Saddam had were intentions and fragments of programs, there was no need for war in March 2003. Thousands of deaths could have been avoided and the dangerous chaos that now pervades the region could have been prevented.

10

The United States Needs a Missile Defense System

The White House

The White House was occupied by George W. Bush, the forty-third president of the United States, when this viewpoint was written. The White House Web site (www.whitehouse.gov) publishes statements on various important policy issues that reflect the views of the incumbent president.

Threats to U.S. security have changed since the Cold War and require a revision of America's defense strategies. The deployment of a missile defense system, capable of intercepting enemy missiles aimed at the United States, is necessary to protect America and its allies. Unlike the United States and the Soviet Union during the Cold War, today hostile states and terrorists are risk-prone and see nuclear arms as weapons of choice, not of last resort. A missile defense system will dissuade these parties from pursuing the development of nuclear weapons by rendering such arms worthless.

Restructuring our defense and deterrence capabilities to correspond to emerging threats remains one of the Administration's highest priorities, and the deployment of missile defenses is an essential component of this broader effort.

A changed security environment

As the [September 11, 2001, terrorist attacks] demonstrated, the security environment is more complex and less predictable than in the past. We face growing threats from weapons of mass destruction (WMD) in the hands of states or non-state actors, threats that range from terrorism to ballistic missiles intended to intimidate and coerce us by holding the U.S. and our friends and allies hostage to WMD attack.

Hostile states, including those that sponsor terrorism, are investing large resources to develop and acquire ballistic missiles of increasing range and sophistication that could be used against the United States and our friends and allies. These same states have chemical, biological, and/or

The White House, "National Policy on Ballistic Missile Defense Fact Sheet," www.whitehouse.gov, May 20, 2003.

nuclear weapons programs. In fact, one of the factors that make long-range ballistic missiles attractive as a delivery vehicle for weapons of mass destruction is that the United States and our allies lack effective defenses against this threat.

The contemporary and emerging missile threat from hostile states is fundamentally different from that of the Cold War and requires a different approach to deterrence and new tools for defense. The strategic logic of the past may not apply to these new threats, and we cannot be wholly dependent on our capability to deter them. Compared to the Soviet Union, their leaderships often are more risk prone. These are leaders that also see WMD as weapons of choice, not of last resort. Weapons of mass destruction are their most lethal means to compensate for our conventional strength and to allow them to pursue their objectives through force, coercion, and intimidation.

The contemporary and emerging missile threat . . . is fundamentally different from that of the Cold War and requires a different approach.

Deterring these threats will be difficult. There are no mutual understandings or reliable lines of communication with these states. Our new adversaries seek to keep us out of their region, leaving them free to support terrorism and to pursue aggression against their neighbors. By their own calculations, these leaders may believe they can do this by holding a few of our cities hostage. Our adversaries seek enough destructive capability to blackmail us from coming to the assistance of our friends who would then become the victims of aggression.

Some states are aggressively pursuing the development of weapons of mass destruction and long-range missiles as a means of coercing the United States and our allies. To deter such threats, we must devalue missiles as tools of extortion and aggression, undermining the confidence of our adversaries that threatening a missile attack would succeed in blackmailing us. In this way, although missile defenses are not a replacement for an offensive response capability, they are an added and critical dimension of contemporary deterrence. Missile defenses will also help to assure allies and friends, and to dissuade countries from pursuing ballistic missiles in the first instance by undermining their military utility.

The National Missile Defense Act of 1999

On July 22, 1999, the National Missile Defense Act of 1999 (Public Law 106-38) was signed into law. This law states, "It is the policy of the United States to deploy as soon as is technologically possible an effective National Missile Defense system capable of defending the territory of the United States against limited ballistic missile attack (whether accidental, unauthorized, or deliberate) with funding subject to the annual authorization of appropriations and the annual appropriation of funds for National Missile Defense." The Administration's program on missile defense is fully consistent with this policy.

At the outset of this Administration, the President [George W. Bush] directed his Administration to examine the full range of available technologies and basing modes for missile defenses that could protect the United States, our deployed forces, and our friends and allies. Our policy is to develop and deploy, at the earliest possible date, ballistic missile defenses drawing on the best technologies available.

The deployment of effective missile defenses is an essential element of the United States' broader efforts to . . . meet the new threats we face.

The Administration has also eliminated the artificial distinction between "national" and "theater" missile defenses.

The defenses we will develop and deploy must be capable of not only defending the United States and our deployed forces, but also friends and allies; The distinction between theater and national defenses was largely a product of the ABM [Anti-Ballistic Missile] Treaty and is outmoded. For example, some of the systems we are pursuing, such as boost-phase defenses, are inherently capable of intercepting missiles of all ranges, blurring the distinction between theater and national defenses; and the terms "theater" and "national" are interchangeable depending on the circumstances, and thus are not a meaningful means of categorizing missile defenses. For example, some of the systems being pursued by the United States to protect deployed forces are capable of defending the entire national territory of some friends and allies, thereby meeting the definition of a "national" missile defense system.

Building on previous missile defense work, . . . the Defense Department has pursued a robust research, development, testing, and evaluation program designed to develop layered defenses capable of intercepting missiles of varying ranges in all phases of flight. The testing regimen employed has become increasingly stressing, and the results of recent tests have been impressive.

Fielding missile defenses

In light of the changed security environment and progress made to date in our development efforts, the United States plans to begin deployment of a set of missile defense capabilities in 2004. These capabilities will serve as a starting point for fielding improved and expanded missile defense capabilities later.

We are pursuing an evolutionary approach to the development and deployment of missile defenses to improve our defenses over time. The United States will not have a final, fixed missile defense architecture. Rather, we will deploy an initial set of capabilities that will evolve to meet the changing threat and to take advantage of technological developments. The composition of missile defenses, to include the number and location of systems deployed, will change over time.

In August 2002, the Administration proposed an evolutionary way ahead for the deployment of missile defenses. The capabilities planned for operational use in 2004 and 2005 will include ground-based interceptors, sea-based interceptors, additional Patriot (PAC-3) units, and sensors based on land, at sea, and in space. In addition, the United States will work with allies to upgrade key early-warning radars as part of our capabilities.

Under our approach, these capabilities may be improved through additional measures such as:

Deployment of additional ground- and sea-based interceptors, and Patriot (PAC-3) units; Initial deployment of the THAAD [Theater High Altitude Area Defense] and Airborne Laser systems; Development of a family of boost-phase and midcourse hit-to-kill interceptors based on sea-, air-, and ground-based platforms; Enhanced sensor capabilities; and Development and testing of space-based defenses.

The Defense Department will begin to implement this approach and will move forward with plans to deploy a set of initial missile defense capabilities beginning in 2004.

Cooperation with friends and allies

Because the threats of the 21st century also endanger our friends and allies around the world, it is essential that we work together to defend against these threats. Missile defense cooperation will be a feature of U.S. relations with close, long-standing allies, and an important means to build new relationships with new friends like Russia. Consistent with these goals:

The U.S. will develop and deploy missile defenses capable of protecting not only the United States and our deployed forces, but also friends and allies; We will also structure the missile defense program in a manner that encourages industrial participation by friends and allies, consistent with overall U.S. national security; and we will also promote international missile defense cooperation, including within bilateral and alliance structures such as NATO [North Atlantic Treaty Organization].

As part of our efforts to deepen missile defense cooperation with friends and allies, the United States will seek to eliminate impediments to such cooperation. We will review existing policies and practices governing technology sharing and cooperation on missile defense, including U.S. export control regulations and statutes, with this aim in mind.

The goal of the Missile Technology Control Regime (MTCR) is to help reduce the global missile threat by curbing the flow of missiles and related technology to proliferators. The MTCR and missile defenses play complementary roles in countering the global missile threat. The United States intends to implement the MTCR in a manner that does not impede missile defense cooperation with friends and allies.

The need to act

The new strategic challenges of the 21st century require us to think differently, but they also require us to act. The deployment of effective missile defenses is an essential element of the United States' broader efforts to transform our defense and deterrence policies and capabilities to meet the new threats we face. Defending the American people against these new threats is the Administration's highest priority.

11

The Missile Defense System Currently Being Developed Will Not Work

Philip E. Coyle

Philip E. Coyle, former assistant secretary for test and evaluation at the Pentagon, is a senior adviser at the Center for Defense Information.

The Bush administration is using an unrealistic timetable for the development of a national missile defense system, which is supposed to intercept missiles aimed at the United States. In its haste to get the system up and running, the Missile Defense Agency is cutting corners, such as reducing the number of tests run on the system, making the tests easier for the system to pass, and purchasing equipment not yet proven to be effective. Deployment plans are also proceeding despite countless technological problems, such as the system's failure to differentiate missiles from decoys. If the missile defense system is deployed in 2004 as promised, it will prove incapable of protecting the United States from incoming missiles.

The clock is ticking. Last December [2002], President George W. Bush announced plans to begin deployment of a strategic nationwide missile defense system at Fort Greely, Alaska, by September 30, 2004. With less than a year left before that deadline, it is clear that the president's decision has drastically changed the priorities in the missile defense program and lowered the bar on the acceptable standards for an effective military system.

If the Bush administration's now anemic testing schedule continues on track, the United States is set to deploy a missile defense system that is simply not up to the job. The ground-based midcourse defense (GMD) system, as it is now called, has not shown that it can hit anything other than missiles whose trajectory and targets have been preprogrammed by missile defense contractors to eliminate the surprise or certainty of battle. Nor has it proven that it can hit a tumbling target, perform at night, or find ways

Philip E. Coyle, "Is Missile Defense on Target?" *Arms Control Today*, vol. 33, October 2003, p. 7.

to counter the decoys and countermeasures that a real enemy would use to throw a defense off track. Tests so far have all been conducted at unrealistically low speeds and altitudes, and it is not clear that the system will be able to track and identify the warhead it is supposed to destroy.

Such criticism is not partisan in nature. Bush's new testing schedule lags not only the comprehensive tests planned by the Clinton administration, but even the testing objectives of Bush's first two years. Indeed, the Pentagon's current missile defense plan marks a radical shift from a half-century of military testing carried out under Republican and Democratic administrations alike.

After Bush's announcement, the missile defense program's priorities immediately switched from challenging and necessary testing to building facilities at Fort Greely and hauling hardware and equipment to Alaska. Since construction began on June 15, 2002, 550 acres have been cleared, at least 620,000 cubic yards of dirt have been removed, 11 buildings have been built, and 25 others refurbished. Six missile silos are to be completed by next February [2004], 10 more by the end of 2005, and as many as 40 in the years to come. Yet, the ability of the missile defense system to carry out its required tasks has barely inched forward.

Before the deployment decision

As envisioned, the GMD system is meant to consist of a set of silo-based interceptors, beginning with six at Fort Greely and four at Vandenberg Air Force Base in California. These interceptors are to carry infrared detectors capable of discriminating enemy warheads from decoys. The system is slated to include a mobile, sea-based X-band radar as well as fixed early warning radars at Shemya, at the end of the Aleutian chain, and at Beale Air Force Base near Sacramento [California], as well as early warning radars in England and Greenland. It also is to use satellites with infrared detectors capable of distinguishing between launches of peaceful rockets and ICBMs [intercontinental ballistic missiles] and discriminating enemy warheads from decoys. Finally, the GMD system is supposed to have a complex battle management command and control system that includes a network of satellites and ground elements extending from Washington, D.C., to Alaska, including Cheyenne Mountain in Colorado and sites in California.

The United States is set to deploy a missile defense system that is simply not up to the job.

In developing a schedule to develop and test the components needed for this system, the president began with a system inherited from his predecessor. The GMD system has more than a passing resemblance to the National Missile Defense (NMD) system planned by President Bill Clinton to protect the United States from attack by long-range ballistic missiles. However, the GMD system is now only the canter-piece of the larger Bush Ballistic Missile Defense System (BMDS), a "layered" system intended to be capable of shooting down missiles in all phases of their flight—boost, midcourse, and terminal—and from platforms based on land, at sea, in aircraft, and in space.

During the first two years of the Bush administration, the Pentagon carried out a testing program that did not depart radically from its predecessor. To be sure, there were some changes. The Bush administration has conducted five flight intercept tests of the GMD system as opposed to three flight intercept tests of the NMD system in the final two years of the Clinton administration. On the other hand, all of the flight intercept tests attempted in the first two years of the Bush administration were quite similar to tests during the Clinton years and did not push the state of the art as strongly as tests either planned or accomplished during the Clinton administration.

Not only does the lack of stressing flight intercept tests undermine military effectiveness, it also weakens public accountability.

The Bush administration has shown some political wisdom in following a cautious script. Year after year, delays in the development program had stretched out the planned milestones, and mounting technical difficulties had shown that this program was no different than any other high-technology military development. It would not be surprising if it took a decade or more to develop an effective military capability. Only six days before the president's deployment decision, the program had experienced yet another dramatic failure when an interceptor "kill vehicle" failed to separate from its rocket booster. To the people doing the actual work, the last thing they expected was an order from the president to move the schedule for deployment to the left.

Testing not accelerated

Bush administration officials such as Lt. Gen. Ronald Kadish, the head of the Missile Defense Agency (MDA), have sought to calm concerns expressed by Congress and the press by saying that the Pentagon would rev up the pace of testing to meet the president's goals. Yet, overall the pace of flight intercept tests and, most importantly the rate of successful flight intercept tests, has stayed about the same. Since the inception of flight intercept tests in October 1999, five successful intercepts have been carried out in eight attempts. That is a rate of about one success every 10 months. At that pace, it could take 10 or 15 years before the GMD system could pass the 20 or 30 developmental tests required before realistic operational testing could be conducted. Developmental tests, especially in the early years of a program, may be heavily scripted with unrealistic or artificial limitations. Operational testing, on the other hand, must be realistic with the systems operated by real soldiers, sailors, airmen, or Marines, as they would be in battle.

Yet, intent on deploying the system in time for the 2004 presidential elections, the Bush administration has sought to act as if the necessary milestones were unnecessary obstacles. Just look at how the Pentagon dealt with problems caused by the unreliable surrogate booster rocket used in the first eight flight intercept tests, as well as delays in the operational, production version needed to launch the "kill vehicle" to collide with incoming missiles in space: it simply cancelled nearly half of the intercept flight tests it had initially outlined. Unable to make the system square with the usual Pentagon definitions of military capable programs, the Department of Defense has dumbed down the requirements for a militarily effective program. Incapable of having key components such as an eagle-eyed X-band radar and flight sensors in place for the "deployment date," the Pentagon is ready to place the system on operational status even without the parts needed for it to be effective.

The problems began with the booster rockets. Booster development and testing alone has taken about three more years than planned. At one point in the schedule, booster development and testing were to have been completed in 2000, but that slipped to 2001 and now 2003. In the meantime, a surrogate rocket booster, a modified Minuteman ICBM used in all of the flight intercepts tests, has been the direct cause of three major failures. So, program officials saw little benefit in risking high profile future tests on that booster. Pentagon officials are now counting on new prototypes from Lockheed Martin and Orbital Sciences Corporation. Both booster designs are likely to have only one intercept attempt each before they are deployed next fall [2004] as part of the GMD system.

Pentagon officials were able to celebrate a rare success in August [2003] when Orbital Sciences successfully launched its booster carrying a mock kill vehicle. . . . But because of the absence of an effective booster, the testing of the overall GMD system has been set back.

Equally significant, some of the remaining flight intercept tests are gradually being downscaled from full flight intercept tests to "radar characterization" tests and other simulations that do not require the interceptor actually to hit its target. For example, two flight intercept tests planned to have been in the remaining months before deployment have been cancelled and replaced by non-intercept, radar characterization tests. Nor is much progress being demonstrated in the ability of the system to discriminate between actual enemy warheads and decoys and countermeasures.

Not only does the lack of stressing flight intercept tests undermine military effectiveness, it also weakens public accountability. Given MDA policy to classify information about these tests, it is difficult for Congress or the press to track, let alone confront, the agency's claims based on non-flight intercept tests, ground tests, or other simulations that do not involve the clear test of whether an interceptor hits its target.

Effectiveness standards

Last December [2002], Secretary of Defense Donald Rumsfeld acknowledged that missile defenses would not be very good at first. The capability would not be defined by the classic military phrase "Interim Operational Capability"—namely something new with proven warfighting worth—but rather capability, as Rumsfeld put it, "with a small 'c'". Nevertheless, he said, even at first this new missile defense would be "better than nothing."

The president's decision to deploy missile defenses is a remarkable example of a new procurement philosophy at the Pentagon called "capability-based acquisition," which means the opposite of what it sounds like. The priority is on acquisition and deployment, not demonstrated, effective warfighting capability. In a sign of the times, last January [2002], Joint Chiefs Chairman Gen. Richard Myers circulated a new draft Instruction on the Joint Capabilities Integration and Development System that officially eliminates military requirements, replaces them with "capabilities," and talks about "crafting capabilities within the art of the possible."

Capability-based acquisition can mean buying new equipment that has not been through realistic operational testing.

In addition to speaking of capability-based acquisition, U.S. defense officials also talk in terms of spiral development or evolutionary acquisition. These terms are used more or less interchangeably and, except for the fact that they all describe an interactive approach for building capability, no one in the Pentagon seems to know what they really mean or how to implement them in practice.

The term "spiral development" originates with Professor Barry Boehm, director of the University of Southern California Center for Software Engineering. In Boehm's model, rigorous testing is needed at each loop in the developmental process. In the Defense Department, however, spiral development is seen as a way to avoid testing and to cut corners.

The traditional Defense Department approach—sometimes called "fly before buy"—is to wait to procure a new military system until it has successfully demonstrated that it can work in realistic operational tests designed to simulate real-world conditions. For major defense acquisition systems, the law prohibits full-rate production until the system has been through realistic operational testing and the results are reported to the secretary of defense and the U.S. Congress. If the added military utility turns out to be only marginal, such systems are usually cancelled.

But major military development programs can take decades and, in an attempt to speed the process, capability-based acquisition was conceived. Capability-based acquisition aims to streamline the process drastically by shortening development time and deciding to fund marginal improvements to military value that might not have been considered worthy of funding in the past.

However, as the president's missile defense decision shows, capability-based acquisition can mean buying new equipment that has not been through realistic operational testing and that offers little or no demonstrated military utility. Neither the GMD system, to be deployed near Fort Greely in Alaska, nor its sea-based adjuncts, to be deployed on Navy ships, has gotten far in its developmental testing; and neither has begun, let alone completed, more stressing and realistic operational tests. That is why the development and testing for both these systems—over the next two years and both before and after initial deployment in 2004—will be so important.

The shift to capability-based acquisition leads to confusion all the way around. For example, a recent General Accounting Office report on the readiness of technology to support missile defense evaluated those technologies against a lesser standard than would be required actually to defend the United States from a realistic threat. . . .

What kind of system will we have?

Assuming the Bush administration goes ahead with deployment, following only one or two more flight intercept tests, what kind of system will we have?

At a Space and Missile Defense Conference last August [2002], Major Gen. John Holly, GMD program director, reportedly said the GMD system would initially have 70 percent of its required capability. Such a claim misleads Congress and the American taxpayer. In 2004, 70 percent of the required engineering and testing will not have been completed, 70 percent of the major system elements required to find and discriminate targets will not be operational, and the GMD system will not have demonstrated the capability to shoot down 70 percent of enemy missiles launched toward the United States. For the GMD system to work in 2004, it requires the MDA getting advance notice from the enemy—say, North Korea. This is because the GMD system has never been tested without enemy target information being provided—and preprogrammed into the system—well in advance of interceptor launch and without an element of surprise. North Korea would probably not be so obliging.

Target discrimination

Since the Union of Concerned Scientists Report on Countermeasures was published in April 2000, the most persistent criticism of the GMD program is that it has not demonstrated that it can deal with even relatively simple countermeasures. . . . Early tests included between one and three balloons that did not resemble the target reentry vehicle in signature, motion, or shape. Tests need to be done with decoys that resemble the target reentry vehicle in convincing ways. To be believable, the GMD program must demonstrate that when a decoy actually resembles the target re-entry vehicle in some way, the Exoatmospheric Kill Vehicle (EKV) can still tell the difference. To do this, at the very least the GMD program needs the combined capabilities of high-quality X-band radars, heat-sensing missile discriminating satellites, and interceptors with target discrimination capabilities as well. Problems continue in all three areas, meaning that if a "capability-based system" is deployed in 2004, it will have essentially no real capability. . . .

A scarecrow

Now, with only a year to go, the pressure is on. But difficulties in the development program and delays in the major elements of the GMD system have made it clear that, if anything is deployed next fall, it will be more of a scarecrow than a realistic or effective missile defense capability.

Accordingly, the president's decision to deploy the GMD system in Alaska by the end of fiscal year 2004 has changed everything but changed nothing. To be sure, it has reordered the priorities for engineers and scientists working in the program, as well as curtailed realistic flight intercept testing and progress in target discrimination. It also has changed the standards of effectiveness that the program must achieve and has led to massive construction at Fort Greely.

The president's decision has also served to illustrate the problems with a capability-based approach to testing. As it is being implemented for missile defense, the new emphasis on capability-based acquisition means buying new equipment that has not been through realistic operational testing and which will have little or no demonstrated military utility in 2004. The Pentagon's most successful development programs, . . . continue to rely on rigorous testing. . . .

So, a choice must be made: Rumsfeld can either meet a political imperative by October 2004 or build a missile defense system that works. But the technical and operational challenges of an effective missile defense system are such that the Pentagon cannot do both.

Organizations to Contact

The editors have compiled the following list of organizations concerned with the issues debated in this book. The descriptions are derived from materials provided by the organizations. All have publications or information available for interested readers. The list was compiled on the date of publication of the present volume; the information provided here may change. Be aware that many organizations take several weeks or longer to respond to inquiries, so allow as much time as possible.

The American Civil Defense Association (TACDA)
PO Box 1057, Starke, FL 32091
(800) 425-5397 • (904) 964-5397 • fax: (904) 964-9641
e-mail: defense@tacda.org • Web site: www.tacda.org

TACDA was established in the early 1960s in an effort to help promote civil defense awareness and disaster preparedness, both in the military and private sector, and to assist citizens in their efforts to prepare for all types of natural and human-made disasters. Publications include the quarterly *Journal of Civil Defense* and the *TACDA Alert* newsletter.

America's Future
7800 Bonhomme Ave., St. Louis, MO 63105
(314) 725-6003 • fax: (314) 721-3373
e-mail: info@americasfuture.net • Web site: www.americasfuture.net

America's Future seeks to educate the public about the importance of the principles upon which the U.S. government is founded and on the value of the free enterprise system. It supports continued U.S. testing of nuclear weapons and their usefulness as a deterrent of war. The group publishes the monthly newsletter *America's Future*.

Arms Control Association (ACA)
1726 M St. NW, Suite 201, Washington, DC 20036
(202) 463-8270 • fax: (202) 463-8273
e-mail: aca@armscontrol.org • Web site: www.armscontrol.org

The Arms Control Association is a nonprofit organization dedicated to promoting public understanding of and support for effective arms control policies. ACA seeks to increase public appreciation of the need to limit arms, reduce international tensions, and promote world peace. It publishes the monthly magazine *Arms Control Today*.

Brookings Institution
1775 Massachusetts Ave. NW, Washington, DC 20036
(202) 797-6000 • fax: (202) 797-6004
e-mail: brookinfo@brook.edu • Web site: www.brookings.org

The institution, founded in 1927, is a think tank that conducts research and education in foreign policy, economics, government, and the social sciences. In 2001 it began America's Response to Terrorism, a project that provides briefings and analysis to the public and which is featured on the center's Web site. Other publications include the quarterly *Brookings Review*, periodic *Policy Briefs*, and books including *Terrorism and U.S. Foreign Policy*.

Carnegie Endowment for International Peace
1779 Massachusetts Ave. NW, Washington, DC 20036
(202) 483-7600 • fax: (202) 483-1840
e-mail: info@ceip.org • Web site: www.ceip.org

The Carnegie Endowment for International Peace conducts research on international affairs and U.S. foreign policy. Issues concerning nuclear weapons and proliferation are often discussed in articles published in its quarterly journal *Foreign Policy*.

Cato Institute
1000 Massachusetts Ave. NW, Washington, DC 20001-5403
(202) 842-0200 • (202) 842-3490
Web site: www.cato.org

The institute is a libertarian public policy research foundation dedicated to peace and limited government intervention in foreign affairs. It publishes numerous reports and periodicals, including *Policy Analysis* and *Cato Policy Review*, both of which discuss U.S. policy in regional conflicts.

Center for Defense Information (CDI)
1779 Massachusetts Ave. NW, Suite 615, Washington, DC 20036
(202) 332-0600 • fax: (202) 462-4559
e-mail: info@cdi.org • Web site: www.cdi.org

CDI is comprised of civilians and former military officers who oppose both excessive expenditures for weapons and policies that increase the danger of war. The center serves as an independent monitor of the military, analyzing spending, policies, weapon systems, and related military issues. It publishes the *Defense Monitor* ten times per year.

Center for Nonproliferation Studies
Monterey Institute for International Studies
460 Pierce St., Monterey, CA 93940
(831) 647-4154 • fax: (831) 647-3519
e-mail: cns@miis.edu • Web site: http://cns.miis.edu

The center researches all aspects of nonproliferation and works to combat the spread of weapons of mass destruction. The center produces research databases and has multiple reports, papers, speeches, and congressional testimony available online. Its main publication is the *Nonproliferation Review*, which is published three times per year.

Federation of American Scientists (FAS)
1717 K St. NW, Suite 209, Washington, DC 20036
(202) 546-3300
Web site: www.fas.org

The federation is a nonprofit organization founded in 1945 as the Federation of Atomic Scientists. Its founders were members of the Manhattan Project, creators of the atom bomb and deeply concerned about the implications of its use for the future of humankind. FAS's strategies include advocacy, briefings with policy makers and the press, public education and outreach, collaboration with civil rights, human rights, and arms control groups, and grassroots organizations. The federation has available on its Web site primary documents, fact sheets, and news reports concerning weapons of mass destruction and missile defense.

Henry L. Stimson Center
11 Dupont Cir. NW, 9th Fl., Washington, DC 20036
(202) 223-5956 • fax: (202) 238-9604
e-mail: info@stimson.org • Web site: www.stimson.org

The Stimson Center is an independent, nonprofit public policy institute committed to finding and promoting innovative solutions to the security challenges confronting the United States and other nations. The center directs the Chemical and Biological Weapons Nonproliferation Project, which serves as a clearinghouse of information related to the monitoring and implementation of the 1993 Chemical Weapons Convention. The center produces occasional papers, reports, handbooks, and books on chemical and biological weapon policy, nuclear policy, and eliminating weapons of mass destruction.

Peace Action
1100 Wayne Ave., Suite 1020, Silver Spring, MD 20910
(301) 565-4050 • fax: (301) 565-0850
e-mail: paprog@igc.org • Web site: www.peace-action.org

Peace Action is a grassroots peace and justice organization that works for policy changes in Congress and the United Nations, as well as state and city legislatures. The national office houses an Organizing Department that promotes education and activism on topics related to peace and disarmament issues. The organization produces a quarterly newsletter and publishes an annual voting record for members of Congress.

Project Ploughshares
Institute of Peace and Conflict Studies, Conrad Grebel College
Waterloo, ON N2L 3G6 Canada
(519) 888-6541 • fax: (519) 885-0806
e-mail: plough@ploughshares.ca • Web site: www.ploughshares.ca

Project Ploughshares promotes disarmament and demilitarization, the peaceful resolution of political conflict, and the pursuit of security based on equity, justice, and a sustainable environment. Public understanding and support for these goals is encouraged through research, education, and development of constructive policy alternatives.

Union of Concerned Scientists (UCS)
2 Brattle Sq., Cambridge, MA 02238
(617) 547-5552 • fax: (617) 864-9405
e-mail: ucs@ucsusa.org • Web site: www.ucsusa.org

UCS is concerned about the impact of advanced technology on society. It supports nuclear arms control as a means to reduce nuclear weapons. Publications include the quarterly *Nucleus* newsletter and reports and briefs concerning nuclear proliferation.

Bibliography

Books

Brian Alexander and Alistair Millar, eds.
Tactical Nuclear Weapons: Emergent Threats in an Evolving Security Environment. Washington, DC: Brassey's, 2003.

Richard Butler
Fatal Choice: Nuclear Weapons and the Illusion of Missile Defense. Boulder, CO: Westview, 2001.

Richard Butler
The Greatest Threat: Iraq, Weapons of Mass Destruction, and the Growing Crisis in Global Security. New York: PublicAffairs, 2000.

Joseph Cirincione et al., eds.
Deadly Arsenals: Tracking Weapons of Mass Destruction. Washington, DC: Carnegie Endowment for International Peace, 2002.

Anthony Cordesman
Strategic Threats and National Missile Defense: Defending the U.S. Homeland. Westport, CT: Praeger, 2002.

Anthony Cordesman
Terrorism, Asymmetric Warfare, and Weapons of Mass Destruction: Defending the U.S. Homeland. Westport, CT: Praeger, 2002.

Michael Creppon
Cooperative Threat Reduction, Missile Defense, and the Nuclear Future. New York: Palgrave MacMillan, 2002.

Sarah J. Diehl and James Clay Moltz
Nuclear Weapons and Nonproliferation: A Reference Handbook. Santa Barbara, CA: ABC-CLIO, 2002.

Harold A. Feiveson
The Nuclear Turning Point: A Blueprint for Deep Cuts and De-Alerting of Nuclear Weapons. Washington, DC: Brookings Institution Press, 1999.

Roger Handberg
Ballistic Missile Defense and the Future of American Security. Westport, CT: Praeger, 2002.

Robert Hutchinson
Weapons of Mass Destruction: The No-Nonsense Guide to Nuclear, Chemical, and Biological Weapons. London: Weidenfeld & Nicolson, 2003.

James M. Lindsay and Michael E. O'Hanlon
Defending America: The Case for Limited National Missile Defense. Washington, DC: Brookings Institution Press, 2001.

Alexander Lennon, ed.
Contemporary Nuclear Debates: Missile Defenses, Arms Control, and Arms Races in the Twenty-first Century. Cambridge, MA: MIT Press, 2002.

Scott D. Sagan and Kenneth N. Waltz
The Spread of Nuclear Weapons: A Debate Renewed. 2nd ed. New York: W.W. Norton, 2003.

Tom Sauer
Nuclear Arms Control: Nuclear Deterrence in the Post–Cold War Period. New York: St. Martin's, 1998.

Paul Shambroom	*Face to Face with the Bomb: Nuclear Reality After the Cold War.* Baltimore: Johns Hopkins University Press, 2003.
Jack Spencer	*The Ballistic Missile Threat Handbook.* Washington, DC: Heritage Foundation, 2000.
Lawrence S. Wittner	*Toward Nuclear Abolition: A History of the World Nuclear Disarmament Movement, 1971–Present.* San Francisco: Stanford University Press, 2002.

Periodicals

Ed Blanche	"Israel's Nuclear Arsenal," *Middle East*, February 2002.
Charles Davis	"Why Deterrence Is Better than Missile Shield," *National Catholic Reporter*, August 10, 2001.
Economist	"Farewell to Armaments: Missiles and Summitry," May 18, 2002.
Economist	"Fission and Confusion: America and the Bomb," March 16, 2002.
John Foster	"Keep the Nuclear Sword Sharp," *Los Angeles Times*, December 27, 2001.
Adam Garfinkle	"Power Play: How to Overthrow Pyongyang—Peacefully," *New Republic*, November 4, 2002.
Jesse Helms	"Bush Was Right to Abandon Treaty," *Los Angeles Times*, December 17, 2001.
Hendrik Hertzberg	"Comment: It's a Deal," *New Yorker*, May 27, 2002.
John Issacs	"Ready, Aim, Fire," *Bulletin of the Atomic Scientists*, July/August 2002.
Richard Lowry	"The Nukes We Need: Adapting Our Arsenal to Today," *National Review*, March 25, 2002.
James P. Lucier	"ABM Now," *Insight on the News*, October 1, 2001.
Steven E. Miller	"The Real Crisis: North Korea's Nuclear Gambit," *Harvard International Review*, Summer 2003.
Morton Mintz	"Hair-Raising Hair Triggers: Terrorists, Nuclear Weapons, and What the Press Hasn't Said," *American Prospect*, December 30, 2002.
Thomas Omestad et al.	"A Balance of Terror," *U.S. News & World Report*, January 27, 2003.
Pat O'Rourke	"No Nukes Turn Pro-Nuke," *American Enterprise*, April 2001.
Thomas Orszag-Land	"Islamic Terrorists and the Russian Mafia," *Contemporary Review*, May 2003.
Robert Scheer	"Real Evildoer? The World's Nuclear Arsenal," *Los Angeles Times*, November 13, 2001.
Johnathan Schell	"The Bomb Is Back," *Sojourners*, November/December 2002.

Jonathan Schell — "The New Nuclear Danger," *Nation*, June 25, 2001.

Science & Government Report — "Components for a Terrorist's 'Dirty Nuke' Can Be Found at Your Local Hospitals, Experts Say," January 15, 2002.

John Swomley — "World Domination via Nuclear Weapons," *Humanist*, September/October 2003.

Time — "Osama's Nuclear Quest: How Long Will It Take Before Al-Qaeda Gets Hold of the Most Dangerous Weapon?" November 12, 2001.

Paul Webster — "Just Like Old Times: Russia's Old Cold Warriors Couldn't Be Happier with Their Country's New Nuclear Weapons Plans," *Bulletin of the Atomic Scientists*, July/August 2003.

Eric Weiner — "Islamabad Dispatch: Trigger Happy," *New Republic*, June 24, 2002.

Kenneth G. Weiss — "The Limits of Diplomacy: Missile Proliferation, Diplomacy, and Defense," *World Affairs*, Winter 2001.

Larry M. Wortzel — "China's Military Build Up and the United States," *Insight on the News*, August 5, 2002.

Internet Sources

Joseph Cirincione — "The Declining Ballistic Missile Threat," Carnegie Endowment for International Peace, April 24, 2003. www.ceip.org.

Joseph Cirincione — "The Kay Contradiction," Carnegie Endowment for International Peace, October 3, 2003. www.ceip. org.

Kurt Gottfried — "A Ticking Nuclear Time Bomb," Union of Concerned Scientists, May 12, 2003. www.ucsusa.org.

David Kay — "Statement by David Kay on the Interim Progress Report on the Activities of the Iraq Survey Group," Central Intelligence Agency, October 2, 2003. www.cia.gov.

Index

nuclear storage facilities, lack of security at, 16–19
nuclear testing, 13–14, 38, 65–66
nuclear waste, 16–19, 27, 40–42
nuclear weapons
  acquisition of by terrorists is likely, 16–19, 49, 61
    con, 20–28
  are a serious threat, 4–9
    con, 10–15
  in Iran, 29–32
  in Iraq, 44–49, 53
    conclusive proof of, not found, 57–59
  make world safer, 10–15
    con, 4–9
  in North Korea, 39, 40–46
  rogue, 19
  in Russia, 6–9, 12
  tactical, 13
  unilateral reduction of, 9–12
  in United States, 4–10, 12, 14–15
  see also weapons of mass destruction

oil embargo, against North Korea, 38, 45
Operation Iraqi Freedom, 52
  see also Iraq, U.S. war against

Pakistan, 20, 22, 24–26, 31, 33–36
Persian Gulf War (1991), 12–13, 15, 32, 51, 53, 57–58
  see also Iraq, U.S. war against
plutonium. *See* weapons-grade plutonium
precision-guided weapons, 13
Putin, Vladimir V., 8–9, 12
Pyongyang (North Korea), 42

Qaddafi, Muammar, 26
al Qaeda, 17–18, 21, 24, 38, 46, 49–51, 53
  see also bin Laden, Osama

radar, early warning, 65
radiation, 8, 16–17, 20–21, 27–28
radioactive material, 16–17
radiological weapons, 13
ricin, 52
Robinson, C. Paul, 10
rogue states, 13, 26
Russia
  is nuclear security threat, 4–9, 12–13
  is U.S. ally, 63
  relations of, with Iran, 29–31
  relations of, with North Korea, 44
  sale of nuclear reactors by, 22, 43
  smuggling nuclear material from, 16–19, 23, 25–26
  see also Soviet Union

safeguards agreement, 32, 39–40, 44
satellites, 65
September 11, 2001, terrorist attacks, 17, 19, 39, 48
  aftermath of, 4, 49, 50–53, 60
  effect of, on India-Pakistan conflict, 24, 36
Serbia, 13
smuggling, of nuclear material, 16–19
Somalia, 47
South Africa, 24
South Korea, 38–41, 43–44, 46
Soviet Union, 61
  dismantling of, 8, 17, 47
  influence of, on North Korea, 39
  see also Russia
Spector, Leonard S., 29
spiral development, 68
Stalin, Joseph, 42
Stockpile Stewardship Program, 14
stockpiling, of nuclear weapons, 4–9, 14–15
suicide bombers, 51
suitcase bombs, 26
Syria, 38

Tajikistan, 18
Taliban, 20, 51
Team Spirit exercises, 39–40, 46
terrorists
  are a nuclear threat, 16–19, 39, 49
    con, 20–28
  attacks by, 43, 49–50
  supported by Saddam Hussein, 48, 51–57
  see also September 11, 2001, terrorist attacks; al Qaeda
testing, nuclear, 13–14, 38, 65–66
theatre missile defense system, 62–63
Turkey, 17–19

unilateral reduction of nuclear weapons
  dangers of, 11–12
  support for, 9–10
United Nations
  Monitoring, Verification and Inspection Commission (UNMOVIC), 32, 59
  sanctions by, 45, 51–53
  Security Council, 45, 48, 51
    Resolution 1441, 53
  weapons inspections by, 13, 31–32, 38–42, 45–46, 48, 51–52, 57–59
United States
  diplomatic failures of, 5, 37–47
  intelligence operations of, 30, 40–41, 58
  is a nuclear threat, 4–9
    con, 10–15